Self-Organisation and Evolution of Social Systems

Self-organisation of social systems can be observed at all levels of biological complexity, from cells to organisms and communities. Although individuals are governed by simple rules, their interactions with each other and their environment leads to complex patterns. *Self-Organisation and Evolution of Social Systems* investigates a broad spectrum of social systems ranging from those of simple single-celled organisms to those of very complex ones, such as humans. It examines groups of all sizes, from small as in certain species of primates, to very large as in some species of fish and social insects.

This book deals with numerous aspects of their social organisation, including group formation, task-division, foraging, dominance interactions, infant protection, language and voting.

It is recommended reading for all academic researchers and professionals interested in the recent progress of this fascinating field.

CHARLOTTE HEMELRIJK is assistant professor of theoretical biology at the University of Groningen.

Self-Organisation and Evolution of Social Systems

Edited by

CHARLOTTE K. HEMELRIJK
University of Groningen

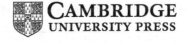

CAMBRIDGE UNIVERSITY PRESS
Cambridge, New York, Melbourne, Madrid, Cape Town,
Singapore, São Paulo, Delhi, Tokyo, Mexico City

Cambridge University Press
The Edinburgh Building, Cambridge CB2 8RU, UK

Published in the United States of America by Cambridge University Press, New York

www.cambridge.org
Information on this title: www.cambridge.org/9781107402560

First published 2005
First paperback edition 2011

A catalogue record for this publication is available from the British Library

ISBN 978-0-521-84655-4 Hardback
ISBN 978-1-107-40256-0 Paperback

Contents

Contributors

Bart de Boer
Artificial Intelligence, University of Groningen, Grote Kruisstraat 2/1, 9752 TS Groningen, the Netherlands

Robin M. Crewe
Department of Entomolgy and Zoology, University of Pretoria, Pretoria 00021, South Africa

J. L. Deneubourg
Unit of Social Ecology, Center for Nonlinear Phenomena and Complex Systems, CP231, Université Libre de Bruxelles, 1050 Brussels, Belgium

C. Detrain
Unit of Social Ecology, Center for Nonlinear Phenomena and Complex Systems, CP231, Université Libre de Bruxelles, 1050 Brussels, Belgium

Serge Galam
Centre de Recherche en Epistémologie Appliquée (CREA), Ecole Polytechnique et CNRS (UMR 7656), 1 rue Descartes, 75005 Paris, France

Charlotte K. Hemelrijk
Theoretical Biology, Centre for Ecological and Evolutionary Studies, University of Groningen, Kerklaan 30, 9751 NN Haren, the Netherlands

Paulien Hogeweg
Theoretical Biology and Bioinformatics Group, Utrecht University, Padualaan 8, 3584 CH Utrecht, the Netherlands

Robin F. A. Moritz
Institut für Zoologie, Martin-Luther-Universität Halle-Wittenberg, Kröllwitzerstrasse 44, 06099 Halle/Saale, Germany

S. C. Nicolis
Unit of Social Ecology, Center for Nonlinear Phenomena and Complex Systems, CP231, Université Libre de Bruxelles, 1050 Brussels, Belgium

Julia K. Parrish
School of Aquatic and Fishery Sciences, Department of Zoology, University of Washington, Seattle, WA 98195, USA

Bernard Thierry
Centre d'Ecologie, Physiologie et Ethologie, Centre National de la Recherche Scientifique UPR 9010, 23 rue Becquerel, 67087 Strasbourg, France

Steven V. Viscido
Northwest Fisheries Science Center, 2725 Montlake Boulevard East, Seattle, WA 98112, USA

Cornelis J. Weijer
Division of Cell and Developmental Biology, Wellcome Trust Biocentre, School of Life Sciences, University of Dundee, Dundee DD1 5EH, UK

David Sloan Wilson
Departments of Biology and Anthropolgy, Binghamton University, Binghamton, NY 13902, USA

Preface

The study of social systems from the perspective of complexity science leads to unusual results that show that, by self-organisation, complex patterns of behaviour may arise from very simple behavioural rules (Schelling, 1978; Camazine *et al.*, 2001). By building these rules into certain computer models we develop a new type of understanding (Braitenberg, 1984; Pfeifer and Scheier, 1999).

This method may be applied to social systems of all kinds and of all organisms. Yet, so far, it has rarely been used among biologists. Moreover, biologists are little aware of the use of this method in the study of social systems in humans.

Therefore, we feel that there is need for a book on social systems of animals and humans from the perspective of complexity science. In order to interest also empirical scientists in this approach, the book contains both empirical papers and theoretical ones.

To realise all this a conference was essential: we organised a five-day conference in the beautiful surroundings of Monte Verità in Switzerland. The authors of the papers of this book were invited speakers at this conference. I wish to thank them for the timely submission of their papers and for their cooperative attitude during refereeing. I am grateful to Paulien Hogeweg, and Bernard Thierry for their useful general comments and to Jens Krause and Hanspeter Kunz for refereeing and to Dan Reid for his work on the index. I am grateful to the Centro Stefano Franscini of the Eidgenössische Technische Hochschule Zürich and the University of Zürich for their liberal financial support.

References

Braitenberg, V. (1984). *Vehicles: Experiments in Synthetic Psychology*. Cambridge, MA: MIT Press.

Camazine, S., Deneubourg, J.-L., Franks, N. R. *et al.* (2001). *Self-Organisation in Biological Systems*. Princeton, NJ: Princeton University Press.

Pfeifer, R. and Scheier, C. (1999). *Understanding Intelligence*. Cambridge, MA: MIT Press.

Schelling, T. C. (1978). *Micromotives and Macrobehavior*. New York: W. W. Norton.

Introduction

CHARLOTTE K. HEMELRIJK
University of Groningen

This book contains a collection of studies of social behaviour that are mainly biologically oriented and are carried out from the perspective of emergent effects and of self-organisation. It brings together papers that show emergent aspects of social behaviour through interaction with the environment in the entire range of organisms (from single-celled organisms via slugs, insects, fish and primates to humans). This book treats the broadest range of organisms as regards self-organisation and social behaviour that has been treated so far in one book. It is only followed by the book by Camazine *et al.* (2001) in which mostly insect societies are emphasised. Most of the papers deal with the direct effect of self-organisation on patterns of social behaviour. We will treat them in increasing order of complexity from slime moulds to humans (Chapters 1–8). A few papers discuss the intricate relationship between evolution and self-organisation (Chapters 9 and 10).

Before treating each of the papers in turn, a few words about self-organisation and emergent effects by interaction with the environment are needed.

Emergent phenomena arise in social systems as a consequence of self-reinforcing effects and of 'locality' of interactions, as explained below. Self-reinforcing effects imply that if an event takes place, it increases the likelihood that it will happen again. An example is population growth. The larger a population gets, the more individuals it contains that can bear new offspring.

Other examples of self-reinforcing effects treated in this book are the cell-clustering mechanism coordinated through waves of cyclic AMP in the slime mould (Chapter 1), the marking and following of trails by ants (Chapter 2), the

Self-Organisation and Evolution of Social Systems, ed. Charlotte K. Hemelrijk.
Published by Cambridge University Press. © Cambridge University Press 2005.

physiologically induced threshold changes for certain activities of honeybees (Chapter 3), the 'winner/loser' effect during competitive interactions (Chapter 5) and the usefulness of certain words compared to others (Chapter 7).

By the 'locality of interactions', we mean that individuals have information about, interact with, and change their environment only as far as it is nearby. This is due to the limitation of their sensory system and cognitive capacity. This locality leads to spatial patterns by self-organisation. For instance, it causes queens of honeybees to be able to suppress nearby workers better than those further off, and this influences their behavioural profiles (Chapter 3); it means that individuals that coordinate only with others nearby show flexible swarming behaviour (Chapter 4), it leads to a certain spatial distribution of individuals of different dominance ranks in groups of animals that compete (Chapter 5) and it leads to biases in voting systems with the majority rule (Chapter 8).

Self-organisation operates on any living organism, independent of its intelligence. However, biologists study self-organisation mainly in species with limited cognitive abilities, such as unicellular organisms (the slime mould) and social insects (ants, bees and wasps) and they are usually not aware of related work on humans by sociologists and linguists. However, that self-organisation is crucial among individuals with a more sophisticated cognition, such as humans, has already been shown in the studies by the economist Schelling in the 1970s (1969, 1971). He was puzzled by the strong segregation of races in certain quarters of a city, such as of New York. Using a cellular automaton, he showed that strong segregation may arise even where very little racism is involved. Related models have been published for the study of, for instance, 'cultural transmission' (Axelrod, 1997), the development of political borders (Cederman, 2002) and the emergence of language (for an overview, see Kirby, 2002). Because of the similarity in approach and since biologists may also learn from studies of human societies, we here publish also a few papers on aspects of societies of humans (Chapters 7 and 8).

As regards evolution, the main message is that because self-organisation produces new patterns of behaviour, it also supplies new characteristics on which selection may operate (Chapters 9 and 10).

The chapters

In the social system of one of the simplest organisms, the slime mould (*Dictyostelium discoideum*) self-organisation operates in the building of a complete organism. Cees Weijer gives an overview of empirical findings and of explanatory models for the occurrence of their aggregation, coordination and fusion

(Chapter 1). When food is plenty, amoebae are single-celled. When food is scarce, amoebae cluster together. This is coordinated through chemical communication. Hungry cells emit a chemical substance, called cyclic AMP. Amoebae are attracted to areas of higher concentration of this substance, and therefore the concentration of cyclic AMP increases more and more. During this aggregation cyclic AMP and cells form spiral waves. Subsequently, amoebae are absorbed into a single body (called a slug) that moves in a coordinated way. Behavioural traits of the slug (such as moving towards the light) arise from the interaction between physical and biological traits of the composing cells and are not separately coded genetically. In the last stage the slug develops a stalk that bears spores from which the next generation grows. Thus, these amazing facts show that self-organisation is a form of design in nature that is very 'cheap' (Pfeifer and Scheier, 1999).

Chemical substances are also important in the coordination of the foraging behaviour of ants. Ants mark their paths to and from food sources with pheromones. At a crossroad they choose the path that is marked the most strongly. Therefore, in the end they communally visit a single (or a few) food source(s) only. The collective 'decision' of the colony to visit a certain food source is an emergent effect of the interaction between ants and their physical environment; when there are two food sources of identical quality and size, by accident one path may be marked more strongly than another. As a consequence, more ants will be attracted to that path and thus, it will be marked more strongly again. In the end only one food source is 'selected' for exploitation. Deneubourg, Nicolis and Detrain (Chapter 2) explain further that the size of a colony affects the 'decision' whether a group exploits a single food source only or several food sources simultaneously. Larger colonies appear to be more likely to concentrate on a single food source than smaller ones, because the degree to which a path becomes marked is greater when the colony is larger (with more ants marking the path).

Intensity of marking and sensitivity is important in honeybees, where it functions in the social organisation of tasks. Moritz and Crewe (Chapter 3) explain that the queen suppresses others pheromonally. Therefore, workers that are further away from the queen suffer less suppression and consequently, they produce more 'queen pheromone'. This influences the tasks they perform (whether foraging or caring for the brood).

Coordination of movement arises not only through trail marking, however. Swarms of birds and fish are beautifully coordinated even without chemical trails and without a leader. Parrish and Viscido (Chapter 4) thoroughly review computer-based models that lead to swarming by self-organisation. They compare this to observational studies of fish.

Swarming consits of coordination of movement, but when a (food) source is reached, competition may prevail. From competitive interactions (dominance interactions) a dominance hierarchy arises. Both in animals and in humans, the effects of victory and defeat in competitive interactions are self-reinforcing: losing/winning an interaction (or match) increases the chance to lose/win the next one. This is called the winner/loser effect (Chase, 1974; Chase et al., 1994). Hemelrijk (Chapter 5) shows in an agent-based model that the tendency to group in combination with such winner/loser effect leads to many emergent patterns of behaviour. For instance, at a high intensity of aggression, a steep hierarchy develops and also a spatial structure with dominant individuals in the centre and subordinates at the periphery. Both reinforce each other and lead to further emergent phenomena, which resemble those found in certain species of primates. It appears that increasing only one parameter in the model (intensity of aggression) causes a switch in the artificial society from characteristics typical of an egalitarian society to those of a despotic one as known from macaques. Thus, many different characteristics of societies may arise from a change in a single internal trait. It follows that, obviously, the genetic inheritance of a social system is then only partial and characteristics of the social system are largely formed through the interactions among the individuals.

In a similar line of thought, Thierry (Chapter 6) points out that not every trait is genetically inherited and shaped by natural selection; many traits are interconnected and may arise as side effects of other traits that are actually shaped by natural selection. He calls such effects pleiotropic. He illustrates them with certain kinds of behaviour of primates, such as infanticide, sexual intervention by youngsters and allo-mothering. Allo-mothering may be a natural tendency of females of all species. That it is not observed in all species may be due to its suppression in some of them. For instance, in societies where aggression is fierce, allo-mothering is impossible, because females restrict the movement of their offspring in order to protect them.

This view of partial genetic determination has also recently been applied to the language ability of humans. Although, traditionally, linguistic investigators considered the expression and understanding of language to be an innate ability, recently investigators have argued that the specifics of language emerge to a large extent from the interactions among individuals. De Boer, for instance, describes that reinforcement through communication causes a kind of vowel system to emerge among artificial agents that initially produce vowels at random (Chapter 7).

In order to make decisions, humans not only communicate directly, they have also invented voting systems (Chapter 8). Galam describes the hierarchical voting

system that is based on majority rule and shows that it leads to very conservative decisions. Suppose individuals may either vote for or against a reform. If an equal number of opinions are pro and contra, the status quo is maintained. This creates a bias against reform. This bias (which operates only if group sizes are even) leads to extremely conservative politics. Consequently, an unexpectedly large initial majority of votes pro reform is needed for actual reform to take place. This is particularly true if the hierarchical voting system contains many layers and the subgroups in which the votes are taken are small.

The interplay of self-organisation and evolution of social behaviour is as yet little explored. We start with two chapters that address the great challenges for future research that are to be found in this area.

Whereas it has usually been believed that complexity restricts the potential evolutionary pathways, David Sloan Wilson emphasises that complexity may also enrich evolutionary potential (Chapter 9). He illustrates the relation between complexity and natural selection with three examples: evolution in fitness landscapes, selection at a group level and selection at the level of the community.

This is worked out in further detail in a highly innovative discussion by Paulien Hogeweg (Chapter 10). She indicates new ways in which self-organisation and natural selection may interact and this interaction may lead to new levels on which selection may act. For instance, interaction among individuals and their environment may lead to spiral waves (such as of chemical components in pre-biotic evolution: Boerlijst and Hogeweg, 1991; Boerlijst et al. 1993). Surprisingly, via selection at the level of the spiral wave, traits may evolve whose immediate effect is disadvantageous, such as slow growth and early death.

References

Axelrod, R. (1997). *The Complexity of Cooperation: Agent-Based Models of Competition and Collaboration*. Princeton, NJ: Princeton University Press.

Boerlijst, M. A. and Hogeweg, P. (1991). Spiral wave structure in pre-biotic evolution: hypercycles stable against parasites. *Physica D* **48**, 17–28.

Boerlijst, M. A., Lamers, M. E. and Hogeweg, P. (1993). Evolutionary consequences of spiral waves in a host–parasitoid system. *Proc. Roy. Soc. London B* **253**, 15–18.

Camazine, S., Deneubourg, J.-L., Franks, N. R. et al. (2001). *Self-Organisation in Biological Systems*. Princeton, NJ: Princeton University Press.

Cederman, L.-A. (2002). Endogenizing geopolitical boundaries with agent-based modeling. *Proc. Natl Acad. Sci. USA* **99**, 7296–7303.

Chase, I. D. (1974). Models of hierarchy formation in animal societies. *Behav. Sci.* **19**, 374–382.

Chase, I. D., Bartelomeo, C. and Dugatkin, L. A. (1994). Aggressive interactions and inter-contest interval: how long do winners keep on winning? *Anim. Behav.* **48**, 393–400.

Kirby, S. (2002). Natural language from artificial life. *Artif. Life* **8**, 185–215.

Pfeifer, R. and Scheier, C. (1999). *Understanding Intelligence.* Cambridge, MA: MIT Press.

Schelling, T. C. (1969). Models of segregation. *Am. Econ. Rev., Papers and Proceedings* **59**, 488–493.

(1971). Dynamic models of segregation. *J. Math. Sociol.* **1**, 143–186.

1

From unicellular to multicellular organisation in the social amoeba *Dictyostelium discoideum*

CORNELIS J. WEIJER
University of Dundee

The development of the social amoeba *Dictyostelium discoideum*

Development of a vertebrate embryo typically involves the generation of millions of cells that differentiate into hundreds of cell types to form a wide variety of different tissues and organs. Some cell types arise and differentiate *in situ* at the right position at the right time of development; however, many cell types have to migrate during development over considerable distances to reach their final destination. One of the best understood mechanisms guiding long-range cell movement is chemotaxis. Chemotactic cell movement is a key mechanism in the multicellular development of the social amoeba *Dictyostelium discoideum*. Its development is in many respects much simpler and more amenable to experimental analysis than that of vertebrates. The cells proliferate in the vegetative stage as single amoebae, which live in the soil and feed on bacteria. When the population size increases, the cells in the centre of the colony will start to starve, and starvation for amino acids acts as a signal for the cells to enter a multicellular developmental phase. Up to 10^5 cells aggregate to form a multicellular aggregate which transforms into a cylindrical slug. The slug migrates under the control of environmental signals such as light and temperature gradients to the soil surface, where low humidity and overhead light trigger the conversion of the slug into a fruiting body. The fruiting body consists of a stalk of dead cells supporting a mass of spores. The spores can under favourable conditions start new colonies, completing the life cycle (Fig. 1.1).

Self-Organisation and Evolution of Social Systems, ed. Charlotte K. Hemelrijk.
Published by Cambridge University Press. © Cambridge University Press 2005.

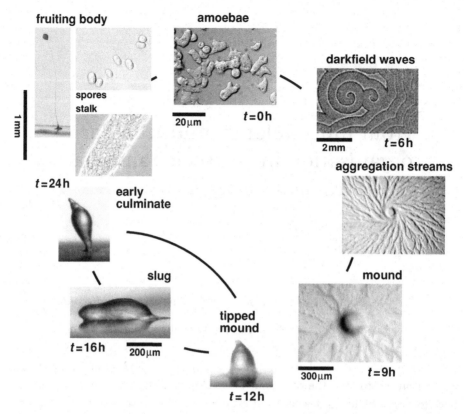

Figure 1.1 The *Dictyostelium discoideum* life cycle. Shown in a clockwise order starting at the top are: vegetative amoebae, darkfield waves as observed during aggregation (they reflect the cells in different phases of the movement cycle in response to cAMP waves), aggregation streams, a top view of a mound with incoming streams, a side view of a tipped mound, a side view of a migrating slug and an early culminate and a fruiting body with on its side high-magnification images of the stalk cells and spores. This developmental cycle is starvation-induced and takes 24 hours at room temperature.

During aggregation the cells start to differentiate into pre-stalk and pre-spore cells that are precursors of the stalk and spore cells in the fruiting body. The pre-spore and pre-stalk cells enter the aggregate in a random temporal order and are distributed in a salt-and-pepper pattern. Then a process of cell sorting takes place, in which the pre-stalk cells move to the top of the aggregate to form a distinct morphological structure, the tip, which guides the movement of all the other cells and is also involved in the control of the phototactic and thermo-tactic response (Kessin, 2001). Since the multicellular phase of the development occurs in the absence of food there is little cell division during development, and the number of cells doubles at most (Weeks and Weijer, 1994). Morphogenesis

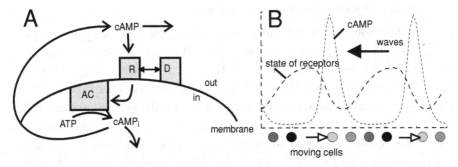

Figure 1.2 (A) Martiel–Goldbeter model for cAMP oscillations. cAMP binds to the receptor (R) and activates the adenylyl cyclase (AC) to produce cAMP in the cell (cAMP $_i$). Part of this cAMP is secreted to the outside (cAMP) where it binds to the receptor again, thus forming a positive feedback loop. Binding of cAMP to the receptor also uncouples the receptor from the adenylyl cyclase (D) resulting in a cessation of cAMP production. Extracellular and intracellular cAMP are being degraded all the time by extracellular and intracellular phosphodiesterase, thus allowing the system to return to a basal state where it be activated again resulting in cAMP oscillations. (B) Scheme showing wave propagation and cell movement. The cAMP wave profile and fraction of active receptors are shown as calculated from the model. Waves propagate from right to left, while cells (arrows and circles) move from left to right. Arrows represents moving cells, black circles resting cells, grey circles cells unable to move as a result of adaptation.

therefore is the result of the precisely orchestrated rearrangement of the differentiating pre-spore and pre-stalk cells in multicellular tissues to form aggregation streams, mounds, slugs and fruiting bodies.

Early aggregation

During development cells communicate over distances of several thousands of cell diameters, using a signal relay system that results in the formation of non-attenuated propagating waves of the chemo-attractant cAMP. Aggregation can be understood to result from three distinct cellular behaviours (Fig. 1.2):

(1) Periodic production and secretion of cAMP by cells in the aggregation centre.

(2) cAMP-induced synthesis and secretion of cAMP (cAMP relay) by surrounding cells, resulting in cAMP waves propagating outward, away from the aggregation centre.

(3) Chemotactic movement in the direction of increasing cAMP, resulting in movement directed towards the aggregation centre, the source of the waves.

Cyclic AMP wave initiation and propagation

A few hours after the initiation of starvation cells become sensitive to cAMP due to the expression of serpentine cell surface cAMP receptors. The cells are now able to synthesise and secrete cAMP in response to a cAMP stimulus, i.e. they become excitable. Binding of cAMP triggers two competing processes, excitation and adaptation. Binding of cAMP results in a fast autocatalytic cAMP-induced cAMP production, mediated by the aggregation stage adenylyl cyclase. Most cAMP is secreted in the extracellular medium, where it diffuses to neighbouring cells (Martiel and Goldbeter, 1987b; Devreotes, 1989). Binding of cAMP also triggers a slower adaptation process, which results in a block of the autocatalytic cAMP production. The cells are now refractory to further cAMP stimulation by signals of similar magnitude. Meanwhile cAMP is degraded continuously by an intracellular phosphodiesterase and a secreted extracellular phosphodiesterase (ePDE). This degradation of cAMP into inactive 5′AMP results in a decrease of the intra- and extracellular cAMP concentrations and the cells be come excitable again (Fig. 1.1). The molecular basis of the complex signalling pathways underlying these excitation and adaptation processes are being rapidly elucidated and are reviewed in detail elsewhere (Parent and Devreotes, 1996). The secreted cAMP diffuses away to activate neighbouring cells, which now in turn start to produce cAMP and stimulate their neighbours. These signals form initially small wave fragments that start to travel through the population of cells. Adaptation ensures the unidirectional propagation of cAMP waves, since cells that have just relayed are refractory to further stimulation by cAMP. The waves will interact and generally form spiral wave centres (Fig. 1.3). There also exists a strong feedback of the cAMP signal on the expression of the components necessary for signal detection and amplification, such as cAMP receptors and adenylylcyclase itself (Gerisch, 1987; Firtel, 1996). As a result the cells become more and more excitable and after a while all enter an oscillatory regime where they are being entrained by the fastest oscillating cells, which make up the aggregation centre.

Chemotactic movement

Cells move by extension of psuedopodia. Vegetative cells move by extending sequential pseudopodia in random directions resulting in a movement pattern resembling a random walk. Aggregation stage cells move up cAMP gradients, as long as the cAMP concentration is rising, by extending psuedopodia in the direction of the cAMP gradient and retracting their trailing rear end. Since the cells are small (~10 μm) compared to the wavelength of the cAMP waves

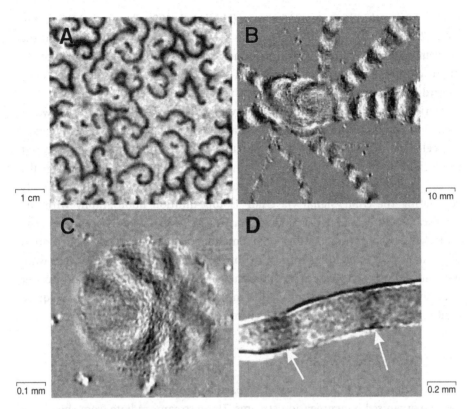

1 cm

10 mm

0.1 mm

0.2 mm

Figure 1.3 Optical density waves at different stages of development. (A) Spiral optical density waves during the early aggregation phase, when the cells are still in a monolayer on agar. (B) Optical density waves in a streaming aggregate. In the body of the aggregate multi-armed spiral waves rotate counter-clockwise throwing off individual wave fronts that propagate down the streams to the periphery of the aggregate. (C) Multi-armed waves in the body of a mound after the streams have reached the aggregate. The waves rotate counter-clockwise directing the clockwise movement of the cells. (D) A slug of strain NP377 migrating from right to left, showing two dark optical-density waves that travel from left to right, indicated by the white arrows.

(~3000 μm), detection of the cAMP gradient results only in small differences (<10%) in the number of occupied cAMP receptors between the front and the back ends of the cell. This small difference in occupied receptors is however faithfully translated in a polarisation of the cell in direction of the gradient. This polarisation process can be visualised at the molecular level by visualising the localised translocation of Pleckstrin homology domain (PH domain) containing proteins such as cytosolic regulator of adenylyl cyclase (CRAC) and protein kinase

B (PKB) during the chemotactic response (Meili *et al.*, 1999; Parent and Devreotes, 1999). The cells stop moving directedly as soon as the cAMP wave passes and the concentration starts to fall (Varnum-Finney *et al.*, 1988). This chemotactic movement response during the rising phase of the cAMP waves results in the periodic inward movement of the cells towards the aggregation centre.

During early aggregation the cAMP waves can be seen as light-scattering waves using low-power darkfield optics (Siegert and Weijer, 1989). Chemotactically moving cells are more elongated than non-moving cells and moving cells scatter more light and appear brighter than groups of non-moving cells. This results in the appearance of dark and light bands in fields of aggregating cells. By correlating the cAMP signal via cAMP isotope-dilution fluorography with the light-scattering waves, it was shown that these waves faithfully represent the underlying propagating cAMP signal (Tomchik and Devreotes, 1981). Most often waves appear as expanding spirals; in some strains they also form target wave patterns. Spiral waves can arise spontaneously in excitable media and do not need autonomously oscillating cells, unlike concentric waves, which require oscillating cells in the aggregation centre.

Aggregation streams

After around 15–20 waves have passed through the population the cells become organised in aggregation streams. These streams radiate from the aggregation centre outward and show a variable degree of branching towards the periphery. Based on theoretical considerations it has been suggested that stream formation results from a deformation of the cAMP wave fronts caused by local variations in cell density in the aggregation territory. A small local accumulation of cells will, due to the autocatalytic nature of the cAMP relay reaction, result in a local increase in the rate of cAMP production. This will locally speed up wave propagation, resulting in the wave front slightly bulging outward in the direction of wave propagation. This will result in the further attraction of cells to this region, increasing the cell density even more (Levine and Reynolds, 1991; Vasiev *et al.*, 1994). Propagating optical density waves can readily be observed in aggregation streams. Most late aggregation centres are organised by spiral waves, which break up into individual wave fronts that propagate down the streams (Fig. 1.3). The wave propagation speed can be as low as 50 μm/min, which implies that the signal propagates around one cell diameter every 10–15 seconds. The cAMP signal hops from cell to cell, as can be visualised by the translocation of CRAC in aggregation streams and mounds (Dormann *et al.*, 2002). Cell movement is still periodic (Rietdorf *et al.*, 1996).

Mounds

Wave propagation patterns

The cells entering the aggregation centre start to pile on top of each other and form a three-dimensional hemispherical structure, the mound. We have visualised propagating optical density waves in the later stages of *Dictyostelium* development (Siegert and Weijer, 1995; Rietdorf *et al.*, 1996) (Fig. 1.3). Continuous measurements of the optical-density waves from aggregation until tip formation showed that the frequency of the waves increases during aggregation while the wave propagation speed slows down (Gross *et al.*, 1976; Siegert and Weijer, 1989; Rietdorf *et al.*, 1996). During early aggregation the period of the signals may be as long as 6–7 min while later in development the period decreases to 1–2 min. Wave propagation speed decreases simultaneously from 600 μm/min to around 50–100 μm/min in aggregation streams and mounds. As a result of this the chemical wavelength decreases from 3000–4000 μm to 50–200 μm. Therefore large spiral cAMP waves initially organise the several-centimetre-large aggregation territories during early aggregation and much smaller spiral waves organise the mound (100–500 μm diameter) during later development. This change in signalling properties is partly due to the cAMP-dependent expression of components of the oscillatory system, described above, as well as to the dispersive properties of this excitable medium (Gerisch *et al.*, 1987; Siegert and Weijer, 1989; Foerster *et al.*, 1990). Experiments using a temperature-sensitive adenylyl cyclase mutant have shown that the optical-density waves in mounds still reflect propagating cAMP waves (Patel *et al.*, 2000).

Cell movement in mounds

The patterns of cell movement observed in mounds are dependent on the geometry of the waves coordinating their behaviour. Cell movement in mounds organised by concentric waves is directed towards the pacemaker centre and slow. In mounds organised by spiral waves, cell movement is counter-rotational to the direction of wave propagation and fast (Rietdorf *et al.*, 1996). The rotational movement of the cells is rather continuous and less periodic than during early aggregation, their movement appears almost fluid-like. The cells still make close cell–cell contacts and the low wave propagation speed suggests that the cells signal only their immediate neighbours. We can follow cAMP-dependent signal transduction in individual cells in aggregates, mounds and slugs by visualising the cAMP-induced translocation of specific signalling molecules tagged with the green fluorescent protein (GFP) from the cytoplasm to the membrane (Dormann *et al.*, 2002).

Slugs

During late aggregation the cells start to differentiate into pre-stalk and pre-spore cells, which arrive in a random order in the mound. Around 25% of the population will form pre-stalk and finally stalk cells and the other 75% forms pre-spore and spore cells. The initial cell type differentiation is linked to which phase of the cell cycle the cells are in at the moment of starvation. Cells that have just divided and are small will become pre-stalk cells, while the cells that were about to divide and are therefore big will become pre-spore cells (Zimmerman and Weijer, 1993; Weeks and Weijer, 1994). As a result of cell differentiation process, the pre-stalk and pre-spore cells start to differ in their signalling and movement properties, which will ultimately result in the sorting out of the pre-stalk cells to form the tip on top of the mound. The tip acts as a signalling centre and will direct the movement of all other cells during slug formation. It controls the behaviour of cells up to hundreds of cell diameters away. The tip has all the properties of an embryonic organiser: when a tip is transplanted into the side of a slug, it will organise the tissue more distal from it to form a secondary slug (Raper, 1940; Rubin and Robertson, 1975). Scattered among the pre-spore cells there is a population of so called anterior-like cells, which are cells that are not yet completely matured pre-stalk cells; these have an important function in cAMP relay in the slug (Sternfeld and David, 1982; Sternfeld, 1992; Bretschneider *et al.*, 1995). Upon culmination they will form parts of the basal disc, upper and lower cup, mechanical structures that attach the spores to the stalk (Sternfeld, 1998). The molecular details of the cell sorting mechanism are still unkown, but may involve differential chemotaxis to cAMP signals (Matsukuma and Durston, 1979) as well as the development of cell type specific differences in motive force arising from differences in the regulation of cytoskeleton and adhesion molecules in pre-stalk and pre-spore cells (Siu and Kamboj, 1990; Springer *et al.*, 1994; Rivero *et al.*, 1996).

We have studied the patterns of cell movement in the slug (Siegert and Weijer, 1992; Abe *et al.*, 1994). Cells at the back of the pre-spore zone move forwards in the direction of slug migration in a periodic fashion. The speed of movement of neighbouring cells is modulated periodically in a similar manner, suggesting that they react to a common periodic signal. As in mounds, cells in slugs do not strictly keep their neighbours; however, all the cells at the back of the slug move on average with slug speed. The cells in the pre-stalk zone show a very different movement pattern. Often their movement is rotational around the long axis of the pre-stalk zone, slightly slanted to the direction of slug migration. This rotational movement is especially strong in the pstO zone (the posterior 95% of the tip, whose cells are normally very motile) when the tip is lifted up from the substrate in the air (Abe *et al.*, 1994). Due to their twisted tracks the speed of movement of the individual pre-stalk cells is greater than the forward movement speed of the slug. This movement pattern can be most easily explained by chemotaxis to a cAMP signal that takes the form of a rotating three-dimensional spiral (scroll) wave in the tip and single planar waves of cAMP in the back of the slug (Siegert and Weijer, 1992). We have shown using model calculations that a difference in oscillation frequency of the cells in the pre-stalk and pre-spore zone can give rise to these wave forms (Bretschneider *et al.*, 1995) (Fig. 1.4). If the pre-stalk cells oscillate faster they can sustain a scroll wave, which twists to form a twisted scroll in the pre-spore zone, a region of lower oscillation frequency. This wave pattern could result from all the cells in the pre-stalk zone relaying the cAMP signal, while only the anterior-like cells, which make up ~10% of the cells, relay the signal in the pre-spore zone (Bretschneider *et al.*, 1995).

Recently we have been able to observe light-scattering waves in the pre-spore zone that propagate from a region behind the tip through the pre-spore zone towards the back. We have shown that the waves originate in the tip; when the tip is cut off from a slug the pre-spore zone stops moving immediately, the waves disappear, and cell movement is disorganised until a new tip is regenerated. The tip on the other hands continues to migrate while producing optical density waves that control its movement. Periodic microinjection of cAMP pulses of the right duration and amplitude can act as a competing signalling centre in the pre-spore zone of the slug and bring all the cells posterior to the site of injection under its control while most of the cells anterior to the site of injection will stay under the control of the tip. This gives additional strong evidence that the tip, the *Dictyostelium* organiser, is a centre of high-amplitude cAMP signalling (Dormann *et al.*, 2000; Dormann and Weijer, 2001).

Culmination

Culmination is the final and most complex transformation that occurs during the *Dictyostelium* developmental cycle. During the final stages of migration of the slug the cells on the top half of the slug slow down their speed of movement while the cells close to the substrate keep on moving. This results in a displacement of the tip to the centre top of the slug to form the 'Mexican hat' stage. During this process the cells in the tip start to form a tube-like structure, by secreting extracellular matrix molecules. This stalk tube, which extends downwards, is the beginning of the stalk. During culmination some of the pre-stalk cells start to move into the stalk tube and move down until they make contact with the substrate. After this has happened they differentiate in mature

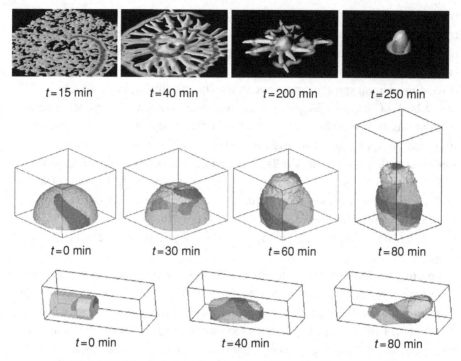

t=15 min t=40 min t=200 min t=250 min

t=0 min t=30 min t=60 min t=80 min

t=0 min t=40 min t=80 min

Figure 1.4 Model calculation of wave propagation and cell movement from aggregation to slug migration using a hydrodynamic model. The top row depicts the aggregation up to the mound stage. The first image starts with the randomly distributed cells which are organised by a spiral wave of cAMP. They form aggregation streams (second and third images) and finally a hemispherical mound (Vasiev *et al.*, 1997a). The middle row shows cell sorting and the formation of a slug. The mound consist of two cells types: 20% pre-stalk cells and 80% pre-spore cells. They are initially randomly mixed. The cAMP waves organises the movement of the cells. The pre-stalk cells are more excitable and move more strongly in response to a cAMP wave. They move towards the centre of the mound and upwards to form the tip. The separation of the cells feeds back on the signal propagation resulting in the formation of a twisted scroll wave. This leads to an intercalation of the cells and an upward extension of the slug (Vasiev and Weijer, 1999). The bottom row shows that a slug organised by a scroll wave can move.

highly vacuolated stalk cells containing stiff cellulose walls. The stalk forms a mechanical structure along which the other cells can move up. During this process more cells enter the stalk tube from the top and the stalk elongates. This process, which has been compared with a reverse fountain, is very complex and requires precisely coordinated cell movement in combination with the precisely controlled differentiation of the amoebae into stalk cells. We have observed that culmination is initiated by a local aggregation of anterior-like cells at the base of the slug at the pre-stalk–pre-spore boundary, where they form a stationary mass of cells. The mass of cells forms by directed aggregation of a selective subclass of cells to this region (Dormann *et al.*, 1996). The majority of the cells follows the tip, moving over this pile, but as a consequence are lifted up in the air. The stationary group of cells eventually forms the basal disc and part of the lower cup of the fruiting body. These cells are characterised by vigorous rotational cell movement. We think it likely that these cells are involved in attracting the cells from the tip downwards to the substrate. However, the molecules by which these cells communicate have not yet been identified. It has been shown that pre-stalk cells are motors for the culmination process. Mutants in several elements of the cytoskeleton fail to form slugs and also fail to form culminants. Restoration of expression of these cytoskeletal functions in pre-stalk cells only is sufficient to restore the process of culmination, showing that pre-stalk cells are the motors in this process (Springer *et al.*, 1994; Rivero *et al.*, 1996; Chen *et al.*, 1998; Noegel and Schleicher, 2000).

Modelling morphogenesis

The development of *Dictyostelium* presents a prime example of the complex interactions and feedbacks that exist between signals generated by cells and their movement responses to these signals and how these interactions result in morphogenesis. A population of *Dictyostelium* cells behaves as a biological excitable medium, in which the cells communicate by propagating waves of cAMP. These waves interact with the dynamics of the medium on at least two timescales. On a short timescale they induce motion and rearrangement of the excitable elements, the cells. On a longer timescale they control the gene expression of signalling molecules, which in turn changes the signalling and movement dynamics of the cells. Since many of these interactions are non-linear it is very difficult to imagine how they will affect development even qualitatively. These interactions are far more complex than those found in most physical or chemical excitable systems and in order to understand them it will be necessary to model these interactions. If we can successfully describe some of the key interactions, it will show that we understand the basic principles involved.

There has been a substantial amount of theoretical work on various aspects of *Dictyostelium* development. Initially many studies were concerned with describing the oscillatory kinetics of cAMP production by single and well-mixed populations of excitable and oscillating cells. In a further development attempts were made to describe the patterns of wave propagation and aggregation behaviour of the cells in two-dimensional models, using continuous, discrete and hybrid models. And more recently it has been attempted to describe the formation of three-dimensional aggregates, mounds, slugs and even the culmination process. I will now briefly review the state of these various models.

The kinetics of the cAMP oscillator was successfully modelled by Goldbeter and colleagues (Martiel and Goldbeter, 1987a; Goldbeter and Martiel, 1988; Halloy *et al.*, 1998). These models in general have three variables, the state of the receptors and the levels of internal and external cAMP. These models although not in agreement with the most recent molecular date still capture the essence of the cAMP oscillator. They can qualitatively describe many of the experimental data on cAMP relay and the development of excitability and transition to an oscillatory regime during development. There have been attempts to model the oscillator based on other assumptions of the molecular mechanisms underlying the cAMP oscillator. They also produce data that compare relatively well with experimental data but are generally more complex (Othmer *et al.*, 1985; Monk and Othmer, 1989; Tang and Othmer, 1994). In a series of pioneering papers Keller and Segel (1970a, b) started to take into account the chemotactic cell movement of the cells in response to cAMP signals, and this approach has been extended by a variety of authors using continuous, discrete and hybrid models (Vasiev *et al.*, 1994; Tang and Othmer, 1995; Aranson *et al.*, 1996; Levine *et al.*, 1996; Van Oss *et al.*, 1996; Dallon and Othmer, 1997; Lauzeral *et al.*, 1997; Dallon and Othmer, 1998; Falcke and Levine, 1998; Halloy *et al.*, 1998; Palsson and Othmer, 2000). Most models are able to obtain aggregation patterns and a stream formation was first analysed theoretically as a streaming instability by Levine and Reynolds (1991).

We have also modelled aggregation stream formation using both discrete and continuous models. We have used the Goldbeter model to describe cAMP kinetics as well as the much simpler Fitzhugh–Naguma model as a generic excitable medium to describe excitable cAMP kinetics in two and three dimensions. We consider the cells either as discrete units that move in a continuous field of chemicals or treat the mass of cells as a composite viscous fluid (Bretschneider *et al.*, 1997, 1999; Vasiev *et al.*, 1997a; Vasiev and Weijer, 1999) that moves in response to the chemotactic gradients created by the cells. Using these descriptions we can model wave initiation during early aggregation, stream and mound formation with all cells having the same properties. By taking into account two different cell types with different signalling and movement properties we can model cell sorting, tip formation and slug migration (Fig. 1.4). To model cell sorting we have to assume that the pre-stalk cells that will sort eventually to the tip of the mound have to develop more effective chemotactive force than pre-spore cells. The mound is initially organised by a scroll wave, which directs all the cells to the centre. The cells that can exert most effective chemotactic forces are able to displace the other cells from the central position where they will be pushed up by the other cells trying to move towards the centre.

The cell sorting will feed back on the signalling patterns in the tipped mound; since pre-stalk and pre-spore cells differ in their excitability, pre-stalk cells as a result of their differentiation are more excitable than pre-spore cells (see above). Cell sorting affects the signalling system in the following way: the collection of fast oscillating pre-stalk cells in the tip leads to an increase in excitability in the tip. This will result in a loss of spiral arms to form a simple scroll wave in the tip (Bretschneider *et al.*, 1997; Vasiev *et al.*, 1997b). The removal of the highly excitable pre-stalk cells from the body of the mound will result in a decrease in local excitability of the pre-spore cell mass and to a conversion of the scroll wave in the tip into a twisted scroll wave in the body of the mound (Bretschneider *et al.*, 1995). This will then direct a twisted counter-rotational cell movement of the cells in the mound. As a result the cells in the mound experience an inward and upward directed chemotactic gradient when they move and this will result in the intercalation of the cells and extension of the mound in the direction of the tip into the air (Vasiev and Weijer, 1999). The structure that forms is a slug, which will fall over and migrate away. These elements can all be caught quite well by any model that describes cells as excitable units and requires the existence of at least two different cell populations which differ in their ability to move in response to a cAMP signal and furthermore differ in their ability to relay the signal.

In an alternative modelling approach, cells are treated as cellular automata. The formalism for most of these models is based on the generalised large Q-Potts model as developed by Glazier and co-workers (Jiang *et al.*, 1998). In this model each cell is represented by an automaton, which is composed of several grid points in space, but has a constant volume on average. Cells can change shape by covering different grid points in space over time, while keeping a constant volume. The changes in grid points covered are governed by a minimisation of the cell surface binding energy between adjacent cells and the substrate coupled to some statistical fluctuations. Chemotaxis is implemented as a bias in this process by a gradient of the chemo-attractant, which results as a preferential extension (movement) in the direction of a chemical gradient (Savill and Hogeweg, 1997). Every cell can have its own internal dynamics of cAMP production and secretion. These models have been used to model rotational cell movement in the mounds and the initial stages of cell sorting but much more impressively to model the formation of slugs and to explain thermotaxis and phototaxis of slugs in response to light and temperature gradients (Savill and Hogeweg, 1997; Maree *et al.*, 1999a, b). It turns out that if it is assumed that light or temperature can locally affect the rate of cAMP production this will result in asymmetry of the cAMP waves, which in turn results in asymmetry of cell movement in response to these waves and a turning towards or away of light and temperature gradients. Finally this model has been used recently to model for the first time the culmination process (Maree and Hogeweg, 2001). The key assumption here is that the stalk gets pushed down in the forming stalk tube through the mass of pre-spore cells as a result of pressure waves developed by cells surrounding the stalk tube on the outside during their attempts to move up chemotactically towards the tip. Although this mechanism has not yet been confirmed experimentally it is an interesting possibility. In order to obtain a complete description of *Dictyostelium* morphogenesis it will be necessary to model the cell type proportioning mechanism, as regards their initial formation and proportioning as well as the stabilisation of these cell types once they have formed and are spatially separated in the slug (Schaap *et al.*, 1996).

   The work described here shows that we are beginning to understand some of the cellular principles involved in the morphogenesis of *Dictyostelium*. It seems most likely that *Dictyostelium* morphogenesis results from the propagation of waves of a chemo-attractant, cAMP, which coordinates a differential chemotactic movement response. The geometry of the signal controls the movement patterns of the cells and therefore the shape of the organism. The proposed mechanism of cell sorting and culmination needs to be further tested by investigation of wave propagation and cell movement patterns in various signalling and cell motility mutants. Integrating the cellular events leading to cell type proportioning and stabilisation of the cells types in the different stages of development will be the next major challenge.

Acknowledgements

   I want to thank Florian Siegert, Jens Rietdorf, Dirk Dormann, Hitesh Patel, Till Bretschneider and Bakhtier Vasiev for their contributions to various aspects of the work described here and the Wellcome Trust and the Biotechnology and Biological Sciences Research Council for financial support.

References

Abe, T., Early, A., Siegert, F., Weijer, C. and Williams, J. (1994). Patterns of cell movement within the *Dictyostelium* slug revealed by cell type-specific, surface labeling of living cells. *Cell* **77**, 687–699.

Aranson, I., Levine, H. and Tsimring, L. (1996). Spiral competition in 3-component excitable media. *Phys. Rev. Lett.* **76**, 1170–1173.

Bretschneider, T., Siegert, F. and Weijer, C. J. (1995). Three-dimensional scroll waves of cAMP could direct cell movement and gene expression in *Dictyostelium* slugs. *Proc. Natl Acad. Sci. USA* **92**, 4387–4391.

Bretschneider, T., Vasiev, B. and Weijer, C. J. (1997). A model for cell movement during *Dictyostelium* mound formation. *J. Theoret. Biol.* **189**, 41.

(1999). A model for *Dictyostelium* slug movement. *J. Theoret. Biol.* **199**, 125–136.

Chen, T. L. L., Wolf, W. A. and Chisholm, R. L. (1998). Cell-type-specific rescue of myosin function during *Dictyostelium* development defines two distinct cell movements required for culmination. *Development* **125**, 3895–3903.

Dallon, J. C. and Othmer, H. G. (1997). A discrete cell model with adaptive signalling for aggregation of *Dictyostelium discoideum*. *Phil. Trans. Roy. Soc. London B* **352**, 391–417.

(1998). A continuum analysis of the chemotatic signal seen by *Dictyostelium discoideum*. *J. Theoret. Biol.* **194**, 461–483.

Devreotes, P. (1989). Cell–cell interactions in *Dictyostelium* development. *Trends Genet.* **5**, 242–245.

Dormann, D. and Weijer, C. J. (2001). Propagating chemoattractant waves coordinate periodic cell movement in *Dictyostelium* slugs. *Development* **128**, 4535–4543.

Dormann, D., Siegert, F. and Weijer, C. J. (1996). Analysis of cell movement during the culmination phase of *Dictyostelium* development. *Development* **122**, 761–769.

Dormann, D., Vasiev, B. and Weijer, C. J. (2000). The control of chemotactic cell movement during *Dictyostelium* morphogenesis. *Phil. Trans. Roy. Soc. London B* **355**, 983–991.

Dormann, D., Weijer, G., Parent, C. A., Devreotes, P. N. and Weijer, C. J. (2002). Visualising PI3 kinase mediated signal transduction during *Dictyostelium* development. *Curr. Biol.* **12**, 1178–1188.

Falcke, M. and Levine, H. (1998). Pattern selection by gene expression in *Dictyostelium discoideum*. *Phys. Rev. Lett.* **80**, 3875–3878.

Firtel, R. A. (1996). Interacting signaling pathways controlling multicellular development in *Dictyostelium*. *Curr. Opin. Genet. Devel.* **6**, 545–554.

Foerster, P., Muller, S. and Hess, B. (1990). Curvature and spiral geometry in aggregation patterns of *Dictyostelium discoideum*. *Development* **109**, 11–16.

Gerisch, G. (1987). Cyclic AMP and other signals controlling cell development and differentiation in *Dictyostelium*. *Annu. Rev. Biochem.* **56**, 853–879.

Gerisch, G., Noegel, A., Schleicher, M., Segall, J. and Wallraff, E. (1987). Signal transduction and chemotaxis in *Dictyostelium discoideum*. *Biol. Chem. Vorg. Hoppe-Seyler Z. Physiol. Chem.* **1987**, 1045–1046.

Goldbeter, A. and Martiel, J. L. (1988). Developmental control of a biological rhythm: the onset of cAMP oscillations in *Dictyostelium* cells. In *From Chemical to Biological Organisation*, ed. M. Markus, S. C. Muller and G. Nicolis. Berlin: Springer-Verlag, pp. 248–254.

Gross, J. D., Peacey, M. J. and Trevan, D. J. (1976). Signal emission and signal propagation during early aggregation in *Dictyostelium discoideum*. *J. Cell Sci.* **22**, 645–656.

Halloy, J., Lauzeral, J. and Goldbeter, A. (1998). Modeling oscillations and waves of cAMP in *Dictyostelium discoideum* cells. *Biophys. Chem.* **72**, 9–19.

Jiang, Y., Levine, H. and Glazier, J. (1998). Possible cooperation of differential adhesion and chemotaxis in mound formation of *Dictyostelium*. *Biophys. J.* **75**, 2615–2625.

Keller, E. F. and Segel, L. A. (1970a). Conflict between positive and negative feedback as an explanation for the initiation of aggregation in slime mould amoebae. *Nature* **227**, 1365–1366.

(1970b). Initiation of slime mold aggregation viewed as an instability. *J. Theoret. Biol.* **26**, 399–415.

Kessin, R. (2001). Dictyostelium. Cambridge: Cambridge University Press.

Lauzeral, J., Halloy, J. and Goldbeter, A. (1997). Desynchronization of cells on the developmental path triggers the formation of spiral waves of cAMP during *Dictyostelium* aggregation. *Proc. Natl Acad. Sci. USA* **94**, 9153–9158.

Levine, H. and Reynolds, W. (1991). Streaming instability of aggregating slime mold amoebae. *Phys. Rev. Lett.* **66**, 2400–2403.

Levine, H., Aranson,.I., Tsimring, L. and Truong, T. V. (1996). Positive genetic feedback governs cAMP spiral wave formation in *Dictyostelium*. *Proc. Natl Acad. Sci. USA* **93**, 6382–6386.

Maree, A. F. M. and Hogeweg, P. (2001). How amoeboids self-organize into a fruiting body: multicellular coordination in *Dictyostelium discoideum*. *Proc. Natl Acad. Sci. USA* **98**, 3879–3883.

Maree, A. F. M., Panfilov, A. V. and Hogeweg, P. (1999a). Migration and thermotaxis of *Dictyostelium discoideum* slugs: a model study. *J. Theoret. Biol.* **199**, 297–309.

(1999b). Phototaxis during the slug stage of *Dictyostelium discoideum*: a model study. *Proc. Roy. Soc. London B* **266**, 1351–1360.

Martiel, J. L. and Goldbeter, A. (1987a). Origin of bursting and birhythmicity in a model for cyclic AMP oscillations in *Dictyostelium* cells. *Lect. Notes Biomath.* **71**, 244–255.

(1987b). A model based on receptor desensitization for cyclic AMP signaling in *Dictyostelium* cells. *Biophys. J.* **52**, 807–828.

Matsukuma, S. and Durston, A. J. (1979). Chemotactic cell sorting in *Dictyostelium discoideum*. *J. Embryol. Exp. Morphol.* **50**, 243–251.

Meili, R., Ellsworth, C., Lee, S. *et al.* (1999). Chemoattractant-mediated transient activation and membrane localization of Akt/PKB is required for efficient chemotaxis to cAMP in *Dictyostelium*. *EMBO J.* **18**, 2092–2105.

Monk, P. B. and Othmer, H. G. (1989). Cyclic AMP oscillations in suspensions of *Dictyostelium discoideum*. *Phil. Trans. Roy. Soc. London B* **323**, 185–224.

Noegel, A. A. and Schleicher, M. (2000). The actin cytoskleleton of *Dictyostelium*: a story told by mutants. *J. Cell Sci.* **113**, 759–766.

Othmer, H. G., Monk, P. B. and Rapp, P. E. (1985). A model for signal relay and adaptation of *Dictyostelium discoideum*. II. Analytical and numerical results. *Math. Biosci.* **77**, 79–139.

Palsson, E. and Othmer, H. G. (2000). A model for individual and collective cell movement in *Dictyostelium discoideum*. *Proc. Natl Acad. Sci. USA* **97**, 10448–10453.

Parent, C. A. and Devreotes, P. N. (1996). Molecular genetics of signal transduction in
Dictyostelium. *Annu. Rev. Biochem.* **65**, 411–440.

(1999). A cell's sense of direction. *Science* **284**, 765–770.

Patel, H., Guo, K. D., Parent, C. *et al.* (2000). A temperature-sensitive adenylyl cyclase
mutant of *Dictyostelium*. *EMBO J.* **19**, 2247–2256.

Raper, K. B. (1940). Pseudoplasmodium formation and organization in *Dictyostelium
discoideum*. *J. Elisha Mitchell Sci. Soc.* **56**, 241–282.

Rietdorf, J., Siegert, F. and Weijer, C. J. (1996). Analysis of optical-density wave
propagation and cell movement during mound formation in *Dictyostelium
discoideum*. *Devel. Biol.* **177**, 427–438.

Rivero, F., Koppel, B., Peracino, B. *et al.* (1996). The role of the cortical cytoskeleton:
F-actin cross-linking proteins protect against osmotic stress, ensure cell size, cell
shape and motility, and contribute to phagocytosis and development. *J. Cell Sci.*
109, 2679–2691.

Rubin, J. and Robertson, A. (1975). The tip of *Dictyostelium discoideum*
pseudoplasmodium as an organizer. *J. Embryol. Exp. Morphol.* **33**, 227–241.

Savill, N. J. and Hogeweg, P. (1997). Modelling morphogenesis: from single cells to
crawling slugs. *J. Theoret. Biol.* **184**, 229–235.

Schaap, P., Tang, Y. H. and Othmer, H. G. (1996). A model for pattern formation in
Dictyostelium discoideum (vol. 60, pg 1, 1996). *Differentiation* **61**, 141–151.

Siegert, F. and Weijer, C. (1989). Digital image processing of optical density wave
propagation in *Dictyostelium discoideum* and analysis of the effects of caffeine and
ammonia. *J. Cell Sci.* **93**, 325–335.

(1992). Three-dimensional scroll waves organize *Dictyostelium* slugs. *Proc. Natl Acad.
Sci. USA* **89**, 6433–6437.

(1995). Spiral and concentric waves organize multicellular *Dictyostelium* mounds.
Curr. Biol. **5**, 937–943.

Siu, C. H. and Kamboj, R. K. (1990). Cell–cell adhesion and morphogenesis in
Dictyostelium discoideum. *Devel. Genet.* **11**, 377–387.

Springer, M. L., Patterson, B. and Spudich, J. A. (1994). Stage-specific requirement for
myosin II during *Dictyostelium* development. *Development* **120**, 2651–2660.

Sternfeld, J. (1992). A study of pstB cells during *Dictyostelium* migration and
culmination reveals a unidirectional cell type conversion process. *W. Roux Arch.
Dev. Biol.* **201**, 354–363.

(1998). The anterior-like cells in *Dictyostelium* are required for the elevation of the
spores during culmination. *Devel. Genes Evol.* **208**, 487–494.

Sternfeld, J. and David, C. N. (1982). Fate and regulation of anterior-like cells in
Dictyostelium slugs. *Devel. Biol.* **93**, 111–118.

Tang, Y. H. and Othmer, H. G. (1994). A G-protein-based model of adaptation in
Dictyostelium discoideum. *Math. Biosci.* **120**, 25–76.

(1995). Excitation, oscillations and wave propagation in a G-protein-based model of
signal transduction in *Dictyostelium discoideum*. *Phil. Trans. Roy. Soc. London B* **349**,
179–195.

Tomchik, K. J. and Devreotes, P. N. (1981). Adenosine 3′,5′-monophosphate waves in *Dictyostelium discoideum*: a demonstration by isotope dilution-fluorography technique. *Science* **212**, 443–446.

Van Oss, C., Panfilov, A. V., Hogeweg, P., Siegert, F. and Weijer, C. J. (1996). Spatial pattern formation during aggregation of the slime mould *Dictyostelium discoideum*. *J. Theoret. Biol.* **181**, 203–213.

Varnum-Finney, B., Schroeder, N. A. and Soll, D. R. (1988). Adaptation in the motility response to cAMP in *Dictyostelium discoideum*. *Cell Motil. Cytoskel.* **9**, 9–16.

Vasiev, B. and Weijer, C. J. (1999). Modeling chemotactic cell sorting during *Dictyostelium discoideum* mound formation. *Biophys. J.* **76**, 595–605.

Vasiev, B. N., Hogeweg, P. and Panfilov, A. V. (1994). Simulation of *Dictyostelium discoideum* aggregation via reaction–diffusion model. *Phys. Rev. Lett.* **73**, 3173–3176.

Vasiev, B., Siegert, F. and Weijer, C. J. (1997a). A hydrodynamic model for *Dictyostelium discoideum* mound formation. *J. Theoret. Biol.* **184**, 441.

(1997b). Multiarmed spirals in excitable media. *Phys. Rev. Lett.* **78**, 2489–2492.

Weeks, G. and Weijer, C. J. (1994). The *Dictyostelium* cell cycle and its relationship to differentiation. (Minireview.) *FEMS Microbiol. Lett.* **124**, 123–130.

Zimmerman, W. and Weijer, C. J. (1993). Analysis of cell cycle progression during the development of *Dictyostelium* and its relationship to differentiation. *Devel. Biol.* **160**, 178–185.

2

Optimality of communication
in self-organised social behaviour

J. L. DENEUBOURG, S. C. NICOLIS AND C. DETRAIN
Université Libre de Bruxelles

Introduction

In animal societies, collective decisions and patterns emerge through self-organised processes, from a variety of interactions among individuals. The rules specifying these interactions are executed using only local information, that is, without reference to the global pattern. Thus collective decisions can be made that, at the individual level, require only limited cognitive abilities and partial knowledge of the environment (Camazine *et al.*, 2001; Hemelrijk, 2002). Simple behavioural rules lead to behavioural flexibility of the society depending on its characteristics (e.g. demography, starvation and kinship) and on its environment (e.g. food distribution and presence of competitors).

Most self-organised decisions and patterns arise as a result of a competition between different sources of information that are amplified through different positive feedbacks. In contrast, negative feedbacks often arise 'automatically' as a result of the system's constraints (e.g. limits on the supply of food, the food reserve and the number of available workers). Amplifying communication is a characteristic of group-living animals (Deneubourg and Goss, 1989; Parrish and Keshet-Edelstein, 1999). One common type of such communication is recruitment to multiple food sources in social arthropods, but also in vertebrates and many others groups. The nature of interactions implied in these phenomena depends on the species and can involve chemical communication and/or physical contacts (Hölldobler and Wilson, 1991; Fitzgerald, 1995; Seeley, 1995; Costa and Louque, 2001; Ruf *et al.*, 2001). Many parameters may influence the patterns of food exploitation as well as foraging efficiency. Indeed, in natural conditions,

Self-Organisation and Evolution of Social Systems, ed. Charlotte K. Hemelrijk.
Published by Cambridge University Press. © Cambridge University Press 2005.

colonies have to choose between several food sources that are not identical: some are close to the nest, some are large, some contain nutrients of higher energetic value.

Many experimental and theoretical studies deal with the link between the collective response and the capacity of single individuals, such as the variables which they are able to assess to tune their communication (Detrain *et al.*, 1999). However, several questions remain open because they cannot be validated easily by experiments. In this respect, models are useful tools to explore the role of each behavioural component on the emergence of collective patterns. Moreover, they give the opportunity to better understand why a behaviour or value of a parameter has been selected and to extrapolate its evolutionary implications.

This paper presents a theoretical analysis of the role of some parameters involved in self-organised collective choices: the number of amplifications or competing resources, the intensity of the communication and the individual sensitivity to a signal. Optimisation is a main question in the study of social organisation and individual decision-making (Oster and Wilson, 1978; Krebs and Davies, 1997) but very few studies deal with the efficiency of communication and information transfer. Therefore, we will investigate how the communication can be optimised to generate the most efficient collective response and how these optimal values of communication depend on the characteristics of the society and of the environment. These questions will be addressed in the context of ants' recruitment by chemical means, known to be associated with foraging mostly but also with defence or nest-moving (Hölldober and Wilson, 1991; Traniello and Robson, 1995). A mathematical model of food recruitment applicable to trail-laying ants is used to perform this analysis.

The model

The model describes the development of the concentration of trail pheromone and as a consequence, the traffic of the ants over each trail. The differential equations describing the time evolution of the concentration of pheromone (c_i) on the trails possess two terms. The first, positive, part reflects the 'birth' of the trail i, $\phi q_i F_i$ and the second, negative, part describes the 'death' of the trail i through progressive disappearance of the pheromone by evaporation, $-\nu c_i$. The flux of foragers from the nest (ϕ) to the trails is related to the colony size. The quantity of pheromone laid on trail i (q_i) is related to the richness of the sources i and ν is the evaporation rate of the pheromone. The function F_i describes the relative attractiveness of trail i over the others. The form taken here is (Deneubourg *et al.*, 1990):

$$F_i = \frac{(k + c_i)^l}{(k + c_1)^l + \cdots + (k + c_s)^l} \qquad i = 1, \ldots, s \qquad (2.1)$$

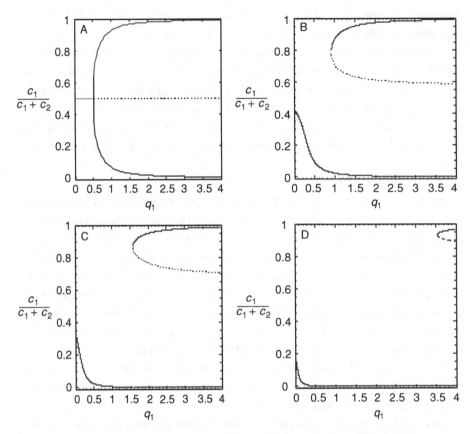

Figure 2.1 Bifurcation diagrams of the steady-state solutions of Eq. (2.1) (for two sources) as a function of q_1: (A) $q_2/q_1 = 1$; (B) $q_2/q_1 = 0.75$; (C) $q_2/q_1 = 0.5$; (D) $q_2/q_1 = 0.25$. Parameter values $k = 6$, $\phi = 0.01$ s^{-1} and $\nu = 1/2400$ s^{-1}.

where s is the number of sources present and k acts as a concentration threshold beyond which the choice of a trail begins to be effective. The parameter l stands for the sensitivity of the process of choice of a particular trail on the pheromonal concentrations c_i present. Large values of l correspond to a deterministic behaviour (close to an all-or-none response). In this paper, most often it will be fixed to a value $l = 2$, drawn from the experiments made in the *Lasius niger* species (Beckers *et al.*, 1992a, 1993). The model equations can be now written in the form

$$\frac{dc_i}{dt} = \phi q F_i - \nu c_i \qquad i = 1, \dots, s \tag{2.2}$$

Figure 2.1 summarises the main results of analytical work previously performed on these equations in the case where two sources are present. It shows the bifurcation diagram of $c_1/(c_1 + c_2)$ with respect to the parameter q_1. As can be seen, when $q_1 = q_2$ (Fig. 2.1A) we have a typical pitchfork bifurcation diagram, meaning that the homogeneous state (equal exploitation of the two sources) becomes unstable at a particular value of the parameter ($q_i = 2\nu k\phi^{-1}$). As q_1 becomes different from q_2, one witnesses the breaking of the pitchfork bifurcation. In particular, for increasing differences between the two food sources (Fig. 2.1B, C, D), the colony is led to exploit preferentially one particular source, since only one stable inhomogeneous solution subsists in a wide region of parameter values. Moreover, in the domain of coexistence of two states, the attraction basin around one of the inhomogeneous solution is greater than that of the other.

In order to sort out the main effects arising from the fluctuations, we used Monte Carlo simulations where the random aspect of the process is automatically incorporated. The simulations are based on the same mechanisms defined in the differential system of Eqs (2.2). We can summarise the different steps of the simulations as follows. When an ant chooses a trail i, it lays a quantity q_i of pheromone that gradually disappears through the evaporation parameter ν. Hence, the probabilities represented by function (2.1) are updated at each simulation step according to the actual pheromone concentrations. The process is repeated for a number of steps sufficient to reach the stationary state, where the total quantity of pheromone over both trails is constant.

The experimental validation of the model has been already carried out in the case where two sources are present (Beckers *et al.*, 1992b; Nicolis and Deneubourg, 1999; Camazine *et al.*, 2001).

This validated model is then used to discuss how the differences in communication and information transfer alter the collective patterns that will emerge.

Optimality of collective choices: the influence of the number of food sources

Let us consider the case where, in natural conditions, ants have to choose between several competing resources. Models give the opportunity to isolate the influence of the number of food sources (*s*) on the food choices of the colony related to trail recruitment.

We consider *s* identical sources (where $q = q_1 = q_2 = \cdots = q_s$). Using (2.1), it can be shown that the behaviour of this system is more complex than the one in which there are only two food sources. Figure 2.2 summarises the behaviour of the model. Keeping all the parameters constant (q, ϕ, ν, k), for $s < s_{c_1}$, we observe stable stationary states in which one food source is preferentially exploited and the others are less but equally exploited. For $s_{c_1} < s < s_{c_2}$, we found two stable stationary states: the previous one and a second state (the homogeneous state) in which all food sources are equally exploited. When $s > s_{c_2}$, the model predicts only one stable stationary state: the homogeneous state. To summarise, for a small number of food sources ($s < s_{c_2}$), the foragers focus on one source, for a

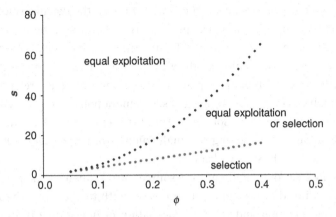

Figure 2.2 Pattern of exploitation in a multiple source situation as a function of the number of sources (s) and ϕ (s^{-1}). Parameter values $k = 6$, $q = 0.1$ and $v = 1/2400$ s^{-1}.

large number ($s > s_{c_2}$), all the sources are equally exploited. Between s_{c_1} and s_{c_2}, both patterns are observed. The randomness of the discoveries will determine the selection of one of the patterns. If by chance one source is discovered a long time before the others, the probability of observing the pattern 'selection' of one source will be high. If most of the sources are discovered simultaneously, we will observe the equal exploitation of the different sources. Keeping s constant, when ϕ (that is related to the colony size) grows, we switch from an equal exploitation of food sources to the state where one source is preferentially exploited. Similarly, when the quantity of pheromone laid on trail q (related to the richness of the sources) is large, one source is also preferentially exploited. The critical values s_{c_1} and s_{c_2} (for $l = 2$) are:

$$s_{c_1} = 2Z \tag{2.3}$$

$$s_{c_2} = 1 + Z^2 \tag{2.4}$$

where $Z = q\Phi(2kv)^{-1}$.

The sensitivity to the trail, the parameter l, also affects the chance of observing the selection of one source: higher values of l will elicit higher s_{c_1} and s_{c_2} values. Moreover, a critical value of $l = 1$ exists for which the model predicts that a colony will never focus on a single source independently of the colony size, the number of food sources or the trail laying intensity.

To summarise, the plasticity in the pattern of choice between several food sources may result without any requirement for qualitative changes in the information exchanged between nestmates nor any change in the individual behaviour of the ants. This plasticity has important consequences when direct competition frequently occurs between colonies. Indeed, the defence is a highly cooperative activity, meaning that the probability of winning a fight increases non-linearly with the number of workers (Franks and Partridge, 1993). Our model suggests that a large colony, able to fight efficiently and exclude competitors at a food site, will more often adopt a pattern where one source is preferentially exploited. A small colony unable in most cases to monopolise a source will tend to scatter the workers on several sources without trying to concentrate its whole foraging force on one site. By doing so, small colonies minimise agonistic interactions and reduce the loss of workers.

Besides colony size, the quality of food sources also influences the pattern of food choice. Knowing that trail intensity increases with food quality, the model predicts that the selection and the monopolisation of one source is automatically favoured when high quality food sources are discovered. At the evolutionary level, the value of the parameters will be selected depending in part upon whether there is a selective advantage in concentrating the colony's efforts on a single site or whether it is better to distribute one's workforce more widely.

Optimality of collective choices: the influence of the recruitment intensity

In this section, we show the existence of an 'optimum' absolute value of q_i in the selection of the richest source and the corresponding choice of a foraging path. Simulations are used to account for the fluctuations inherent to the trail recruitment process. The following results correspond to the situation where two sources are simultaneously offered to the colony. We study the influence of the absolute values of q_1 and q_2 on the selection rate for a given colony size and ratio q_2/q_1. The percentage of simulations leading to the selection of the richest source, R, is the index of efficiency. As seen in Fig. 2.3, there exists an optimised value of q_1 (and thus of q_2) for which the selection of the richest source reaches a maximum at the stationary state. The maximum is higher if the difference (ratio q_2/q_1) between the two sources is larger. This can be intuitively understood since the competition is less marked as the increasing difference between sources leads to less marked competition between trails (inducing the selection of the richest source). Indeed higher differences in trail modulation according to the food quality imply a higher determinism in the choice of the richest source.

We also see that, for increasing values of the flux parameter, the maximum is shifted to smaller absolute values of q_1. The optimal value is always bigger for high values of ϕ and small values of q_1. This shows that large colonies are capable of reaching a high selection rate with small values of q. These results mean that the optimised selection of a trail leading to the richest source is not

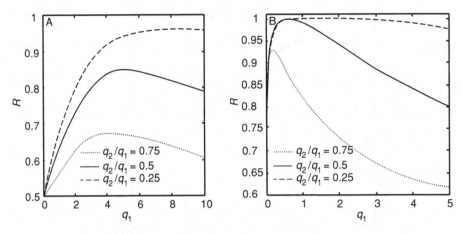

Figure 2.3 Selection rate (ratio of the frequencies (2.1) at the end of the process) versus parameter q_1 for different values of q_2/q_1 with (A) $\phi = 1/600$ s^{-1} and (B) $\phi = 1/10$ s^{-1}. Parameter values are $k = 6$ and $\nu = 1/2400$ s^{-1}.

only due to the relative modulation of trail-laying according to food quality (q_2/q_1) but also to the intrinsic capability of individuals to lay a certain quantity q of trail pheromone. In other words, ants from small colonies have to lay large quantities of trail pheromone to reach a good selection rate while individuals from large colonies can lay smaller quantities per passage and reach a better global selection rate.

It is well known that trail recruitment in ants mainly occurs in large societies. Different hypotheses have been formulated to explain the positive correlation between cooperativity through trail recruitment and colony size (Beckers *et al.*, 1989; Hölldobler and Wilson, 1991; Anderson and McShea 2001). Our results provide further insights on this matter by showing that large numbers of trail-laying ants enhance the efficiency of collective choices.

Optimality of collective choices: the influence of the sensitivity to the trail

The parameter l stands for the sensitivity of the process of choice between i trails of pheromonal concentrations c_i. There is a value of the parameter l for which the selection is optimised (Fig. 2.4.). It should be noted that the l values, which optimise the selection, are between 1.9 and 2.6 (this range includes the experimental value of the parameter for the species *Lasius niger*, $l \approx 2$). Moreover, it can be shown that if we decrease the flux of individuals, the maximum is shifted to higher values of l, suggesting that if a colony possesses

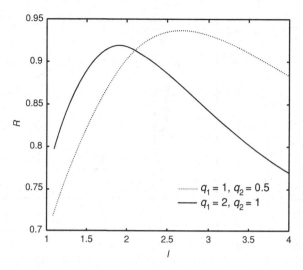

Figure 2.4 Selection rate (R) versus parameter l for $q_2/q_1 = 0.5$ for two different absolute values of q_1 and q_2. Parameter values are $\phi = 1/10 \text{ s}^{-1}$, $k = 6$ and $\nu = 1/2400 \text{ s}^{-1}$.

a small number of individuals, the ants need to have a more deterministic behaviour.

Discussion

The results above demonstrate that changes in the dynamics of information transfer, environmental and social parameters can be responsible for shifts between different collective responses. By increasing the number of sources in competition or by decreasing the number of workers, the colony shifts from a heterogeneous exploitation to an equal exploitation of all sources. The trail intensity (q) and the sensitivity to the trail (l) also act upon this shift with large values of both parameters favouring the heterogeneous exploitation of the environment.

We show the existence of a quantity of laid pheromone and a sensitivity for which the foraging efficiency reaches a maximum, whatever qualitative differences between the two sources might be. Moreover, in terms of colony size, the model shows that large colonies easily focus on the richest source, this selection being sharper if the individuals lay small quantities of pheromone and respond to the trail in a more deterministic way. One should also notice that even for optimised values of communication (q and l), small colonies always perform less efficient food retrieval in terms of energetic return. In other words, small-sized colonies seem less able to take advantage of trail recruitment properties than large ones.

From a stochastic point of view, the quantity of pheromone q and the parameter l have similar effects. Indeed, higher values of both parameters lead to more deterministic behaviours of the ants. The existence of an optimal value for both q and l show that there is a level of noise that maximises the collective response in terms of efficiency and selection of the most rewarding site.

Selected parameter values of recruitment enable animal societies to respond adaptively to the diversity of the environment, despite some simplicity of decision rules at the individual level. It is rather trivial to claim that species-specific parameter values have been selected as trade-off responses to multiple and sometimes opposite constraints. For example, for a small colony, intercolonial competition contributes to selecting low values of trail sensitivity while, by contrast, the optimal exploitation of the most rewarding sources favours high sensitivity values. As we cannot experimentally disentangle these different selective effects, modelling gives us the opportunity to isolate and assess their respective contributions to the shaping of communication.

Results obtained in the work described in this paper in the specific biological context of food recruitment can be generalised to other decision processes involving different competing options (Camazine and Sneyd, 1991; Seeley et al., 1991; Visscher and Camazine, 1999; Camazine et al., 2001; Hemelrijk, 2002). Recruitment systems are used for others purposes such as nest defence or swarming (Hölldobler and Wilson, 1990). Moreover, recruitment has also been shown in numerous gregarious species such as social caterpillars (Fitzgerald, 1995), or vertebrates such as Norway rats (Galef and Buckley, 1996) and naked mole rats (Judd and Sherman, 1996). Furthermore, aggregation can be viewed as a result of the competition between different attractive sites. Aggregation can be described by similar mathematical models when individuals of a colony have the choice between different relative attractive sites to aggregate themselves (Rivault et al., 1999; Lioni et al., 2001; Amé et al., unpubl. data). It can therefore be expected that since the mechanisms underlying all phenomena implying competition are similar to recruitment, the same kind of collective plasticity and optimised value of amplification could be observed.

Acknowledgements

This study was supported by the Belgian Fund for Joint Basic Research (grant no. 2.4510.01). C. Detrain and J. L. Deneubourg are research associates from the Belgian National Fund for Scientific Research. S. C. Nicolis would thank the

Action de Recherche Concertée and the Fondation David et Alice Van Buuren for its support.

References

Anderson, C. and McShea, D. C. (2001). Individual versus social complexity, with particular reference to ant colonies. *Biol. Rev.* **76**, 211–237.

Beckers, R., Goss, S., Deneubourg, J. L. and Pasteels, J. M. (1989). Colony size, communication and ant foraging strategy. *Psyche* **96**, 239–256.

Beckers, R., Deneubourg, J. L. and Goss, S. (1992a). Trails and U-turns in the selection of a path by the ant *Lasius niger*. *J. Theoret. Biol.* **159**, 397–415.

(1992b). Trail laying behavior during food recruitment in the ant *Lasius niger* (L.). *Insectes Soc.* **39**, 59–72.

(1993). Modulation of trail laying in the ant *Lasius niger* (Hymenoptera: Formicidae) and its role in the collective selection of a food source. *J. Insect Behav.* **6**, 751–759.

Camazine, S. and Sneyd, J. (1991). A model of collective nectar source selection by honeybees: self-organization through simple rules. *J. Theoret. Biol.* **149**, 547–571.

Camazine, S., Deneubourg, J. L., Franks, N. R. *et al.* (2001). *Self-Organisation in Biological Systems*. Princeton, NJ: Princeton University Press.

Costa, J. T. and Louque, R. W. (2001). Group foraging and trail following behavior of the red-headed pine sawfly *Neodiprion lecontei* (Fitch) (Hymenoptera: Symphyta: Diprionidae). *Ann. Entomol. Soc. America* **94**, 480–489.

Deneubourg, J. L. and Goss, S. (1989). Collective patterns and decision-making. *Ethol. Ecol. Evol.* **1**, 295–311.

Deneubourg, J. L., Aron, S., Goss, S. and Pasteels, J. M. (1990). The self-organizing exploratory pattern of the Argentine ant. *J. Insect Behav.* **3**, 159–168.

Detrain, C., Deneubourg, J. L. and Pasteels, J. M. (1999). *Information Processing in Social Insects*. Basel: Birkhäuser Verlag.

Fitzgerald, T. D. (1995). *The Tent Caterpillars*. Ithaca, NY: Cornell University Press.

Franks, N. R. and Partridge, L.C. (1993). Lanchester battles and the evolution of combat in ants. *Anim. Behav.* **45**, 197–199.

Galef, B. G. Jr and Buckley, L. L. (1996). Use of foraging trails by Norway rats. *Anim. Behav.* **52**, 765–771.

Hemelrijk, C. K. (2002). Understanding social behaviour with the help of complexity science. *Ethology* **108**, 655–671.

Hölldobler, B. and Wilson, E. O. (1991). *The Ants*. Cambridge, MA: Harvard University Press.

Judd, T. and Sherman, P. (1996). Naked mole rats recruit colony mates to food source. *Anim. Behav.* **52**, 957–969.

Krebs, J. R. and Davies, N. B. (1997). *Behavioural Ecology: An Evolutionary Approach*. Oxford: Blackwell Scientific Publications.

Lioni, A., Sauwens, C., Theraulaz, G. and Deneubourg, J. L. (2001). Chain formation in *Oecophylla longinoda*. *J. Insect Behav.* **14**, 679–696.

Nicolis, S. C. and Deneubourg, J. L. (1999). Emerging patterns and food recruitments in ants: an analytical study. *J. Theoret. Biol.* **198**, 575–592.

Oster, G. F. and Wilson, E. O. (1978). *Caste and Ecology in Social Insects.* Princeton, NJ: Princeton University Press.

Parrish, J. and Keshet-Edelstein, L. (1999). Complexity, pattern, and evolutionary trade-offs in animal aggregation. *Science* **284**, 99–101.

Rivault, C., Theraulaz, G., Cloarec, A. and Deneubourg, J. L. (1999). *Auto-organization et Reconnaissance Coloniale: Le modèle de l'Agrégation des Blattes.* Albi: Actes Colloques Insectes Sociaux Section française.

Ruf, C., Costa, J. T. and Fiedler, K. (2001). Trail-based communication in social caterpillars of *Eriogaster lanestris* (Lepidoptera: Lasiocampidae). *J. Insect Behav.* **14**, 231–245.

Seeley, T. D. (1995). *The Wisdom of the Hive.* Cambridge, MA: Harvard University Press.

Seeley, T. D., Camazine, S. and Sneyd J. (1991). Collective decision-making in honeybees: how colonies choose among nectar sources. *Behav. Ecol. Sociobiol.* **28**, 277–290.

Traniello, S. K. and Robson, J. F. A. (1995). Trail and territorial pheromones in the social insects. In *The Chemical Ecology of Insects*, vol. 2, ed. W. J. Bell and R. Cardé. London: Chapman and Hall, pp. 241–285.

Visscher, P. K. and Camazine, S. (1999). Collective decisions & cognition in bees. *Nature* **397**, 400.

3

The interplay of intracolonial genotypic variance and self-organisation of dominance hierarchies in honeybees

ROBIN F. A. MORITZ
Martin-Luther-Universität Halle-Wittenberg

ROBIN M. CREWE
University of Pretoria

Multiple mating in social insects

Multiple mating of females (polyandry) is a rare phenomenon in social hymenoptera (Strassmann, 2001). The adaptive value of single mating seems obvious: females should mate with as few males as possible to minimise predation risk during mating, the energy costs involved in mating and the chance of contracting a disease. Most importantly, polyandry nullifies the benefits of male haploidy for the inclusive fitness of the sterile workers in the colony. Multiple mating dramatically reduces the intracolonial relatedness (Boomsma and Ratnieks, 1996) and hence reduces the force of the arguments of kin selection theory (Hamilton 1964a, b), because the high intracolonial genotypic diversity creates an extreme potential for conflict among the nest members. Fourteen evolutionary rescue hypotheses have been identified to explain the potential benefits of polyandry in spite of the additional mating costs (Crozier and Fjerdingstad, 2001).

Although considerable effort has been expended to explain the evolution of polyandry, the consequences of polyandry for the organisation of the society have received less attention. The honeybees (*Apis* spp.) may be an exception in this regard. This is primarily due to a relatively large research community working on *Apis* because of its economic significance. The knowledge accumulated on the biology of *Apis* exceeds that of other social insects by far. The other

Self-Organisation and Evolution of Social Systems, ed. Charlotte K. Hemelrijk.
Published by Cambridge University Press. © Cambridge University Press 2005.

rather fortunate property is the extreme degree of polyandry in the honeybee (Palmer and Oldroyd, 2000). Multiple mating in *Apis* can exceed 50 drones
per queen (Moritz *et al.*, 1995, Palmer and Oldroyd, 2001). This makes the honeybee system an ideal one for research on the impact of polyandry on social
behaviour.

The sequence of mating behaviour is best described for the Western honeybee *Apis mellifera*. Virgin queens conduct multiple nuptial flights to so-called
drone congregation areas (Alber *et al.*, 1955). In flight they mate with a variable
number of males representing a random sample of the drone population. Insuf-
ficiently mated queens conduct repeated flights until they have mated with a
sufficient number of drones (Woyke, 1960). It appears that the number of matings is an important signal used by the queen to initiate oviposition (Schlüns
et al., 2001; but see Tarpy and Page, 2000). Once the queen has commenced
egg-laying, she will not mate again, and successively depletes the semen stored
in the spermatheca to fertilise her eggs destined to produce female offspring.
Depending on the origin of the sperm, the resulting female will belong to one
of the various subfamilies represented in the stored semen. In principle this
mating strategy sets the stage for a rather unpredictable genotypic composition
of the colony. The unpredictability of sperm use is further enhanced because the
sperm from each sire is not equally represented in the spermatheca, and the
various patrilines will show unequal frequencies. Although there is no sperm
clumping as claimed in some older publications (Taber, 1955), the distribution
of sperm in the spermatheca is not completely homogeneous (Haberl and Tautz,
1998), and unequal sperm usage may occur (Page, 1986). Nevertheless, the genotypic composition of the honeybee colony is mainly characterized by two major
factors: its complexity and its unpredictability, the one setting the stage for
conflict among subfamilies and the other a large variance for any genetically
determined behavioural traits which may potentially affect colony efficiency.

Regulation of dominance hierarchies

In spite of the high conflict potential resulting from polyandry, actual
conflict is rare in the honeybee colony. The queen is usually the only reproductive
female in the colony of the honeybee. She ensures her reproductive status by producing a suite of queen pheromones, which suppress reproduction in workers.
In addition, the worker police (the removal of worker laid eggs by other workers:
Ratnieks, 1988) prevent successful worker reproduction which is highly adaptive
under polyandry. Under queenless conditions however, workers can activate their
ovaries and worker policing breaks down. This process has been best studied in
the Cape honeybee (*Apis mellifera capensis*). Workers can activate their ovaries and

produce queen pheromones as soon as the pheromonal suppression by the queen relaxes (Wossler, 2002). This occurs typically after a phase of strong intracolonial selection during which only very few workers of specific subfamilies develop into pseudoqueens (Moritz *et al.*, 1996). These pseudoqueens can release and prime the same behaviours and processes as real queens (e.g. attract workers to surround the queen (retinue behaviour), suppress the ovary activation of others). There is a strong genetic variance component for this trait among the workers of a colony (Moritz and Hillesheim, 1985). The results of this intracolonial selection process are extreme, since the differences in reproductive success are huge. In the end only very few workers monopolise the resources of the colony at the expense of the other workers which do not reproduce. It is perhaps the most extreme case of division of labour among workers where only very few specialise in reproduction. Because the phenotypes are so extremely different, reproductive division of labour among workers serves as an excellent example for illustrating genetic effects on the one hand and self-organised processes on the other. Regulation of worker reproduction is understood in detail (Neumann and Moritz, 2002) and can be explained including both genetic variance and self-organisation processes similar to classical reaction–diffusion models (Turing, 1952).

A self-organisation model on mandibular gland pheromone secretion

The classical queen pheromones that are composed of a bouquet of fatty acids secreted in the mandibular glands (Winston and Slessor, 1992, 1998) appear to be involved in the regulation of worker reproduction (Moritz *et al.*, 2000). Freshly emerged workers produce very little of the mandibular gland secretions (Simon *et al.*, 2001), but with increasing age the amount of fatty acids produced, increases. In dominant workers the fatty acid secretion is more queen-like with 9-oxo-2-decenoic acid (9-ODA), the 'queen substance' (Butler, 1959; Butler *et al.*, 1962), being the dominant compound. In subordinate workers a different component of the biosynthetic pathway of fatty acids is emphasised. The critical chemical difference between the major secretory products of queens and workers is the position of a single hydroxyl group (Plettner *et al.*, 1996, 1998) (Fig. 3.1). The development of a queen-like signal in a worker can be suppressed by exogenously applied queen substance. There is an individual suppression threshold for each worker. Workers exposed to queen substance (9-ODA) levels exceeding their threshold do not develop a queen-like pheromone mandibular gland secretion (Moritz *et al.*, 2000). If two freshly emerged workers are kept in pairs, they appear to compete for the strongest signal. Eventually one individual becomes dominant and will produce a secretion with more queen pheromone thereby suppressing the production of the queen substance in the

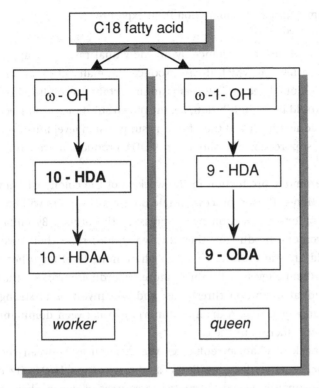

Figure 3.1 Biosynthetic pathway of fatty acids in the mandibular gland secretions of honeybee workers. 10-HDA, 10-hydroxy-(E)2-decenoic acid; 10-HDAA, 10-hydroxy-decanoic acid; 9-HDA, 9-hydroxy-(E)2-decenoic acid; 9-ODA, 9-oxo-(E)2-decenoic acid. Dominant compounds in bold.

other. The dominance hierarchy is settled three days after emergence (Moritz *et al.*, 2003). A simple regulatory rule based on two hypothetical mechanisms can be used to explain this phenomenon, based on pheromone perception and production.

Mechanism 1: variable suppression threshold for levels of queen pheromone exposure

Workers are not suppressed by being exposed to levels of queen pheromone lower than the worker's suppression threshold. Unsuppressed workers will increase their own production of queen pheromone up to their individual genotypically set physiological limit. The suppression threshold is however not a constant but depends on the amount of self produced 9-ODA. If the surrounding 9-ODA concentration is higher than the suppression threshold level, the production of 9-ODA will either not be initiated or will decrease and the threshold for suppression will also decrease.

Mechanism 2: lack of self-inhibition from exposure
to self-produced 9-ODA

Production of queen substance by an individual raises its suppression threshold above the level at which it can produce the material or switches off the inhibition threshold detector. This seems an important precondition because otherwise there would be self-inhibition, i.e. the queen substance produced must not inhibit the producer itself and therefore the suppression level must be raised accordingly. Thus suppression threshold and 9-ODA production are closely correlated.

The queen pheromone production in the workers of the colony will now follow a typical reaction–diffusion process. Single dominant workers will enhance their queen pheromone production by suppressing the others. By enhancing their queen pheromone production they do two things: raise their own suppression threshold and raise the local queen pheromone level for other workers. The new pheromone levels will inhibit more subordinate workers that will lower their individual inhibition thresholds, and will invest more strongly in the worker substance pathway. A distinct dimorphism between dominant and subordinate workers emerges in the colony.

A second feedback mechanism enhances the differences between the two worker types. Dominant workers avoid the suppressive signals (Moritz *et al.*, 2000) whereas the subordinates are attracted to sources of queen pheromones (Fig. 3.2). This leads to a spatial separation of dominant workers surrounded by subordinate ones. Moreover the dominant workers are often surrounded by a retinue of subordinate workers.

The impact of multiple mating

Even given all workers had an identical genotype, the self-organisation mechanism in itself would be sufficient to explain the presence of few dominant and a large number of subordinate workers. However, due to multiple mating the genotypic colony composition consists of many patrilines. Since the development of a queen-like signal has a strong genetic variance component, dominant workers are not selected at random, but workers of specific patrilines will develop into pseudoqueens whereas others will remain sterile. This has profound consequences on establishing dominance hierarchies, and in turn has significant consequences for the composition of the colony with a dynamically changing pattern of subfamily composition over time. Such intracolonial selection of subfamilies can be a major force in determining patriline composition in queenless colonies of the Cape honeybee. Moritz *et al.* (1996) showed that frequencies of previously rare subfamilies can dominate after queen loss.

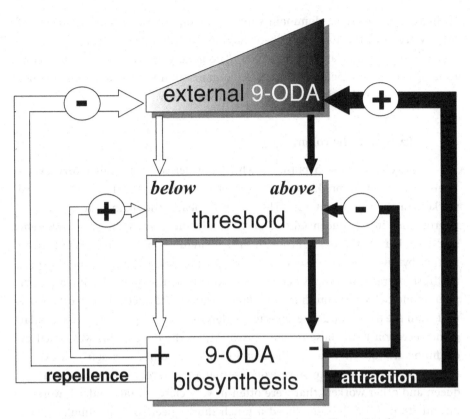

Figure 3.2 Hypothetical schematic feedback-loop system illustrating the
interactions between queen substance biosynthesis and the inhibition threshold.
A receptor detects the external 9-ODA level, which is either above or below the
individual inhibition threshold. Suppression (black arrows, right pathway): if 9-ODA
is above the threshold level, the worker biosynthetic pathway is more strongly
emphasised. This results in reduced 9-ODA production. The reduction in internal
9-ODA lowers the individual threshold level even further (−), thereby closing the
negative feedback loop. These workers are suppressed until they perceive external
9-ODA levels that are lower than their individual threshold. Workers using this
pathway are attracted to 9-ODA sources and external 9-ODA levels perceived by the
worker increase. Dominance (white arrows, left pathway): If external 9-ODA levels
are below the threshold, the queen-like biosynthetic pathway is activated, and
the workers produce mandibular gland secretion with more 9-ODA. The high
internal 9-ODA level raises the inhibition threshold (+), thus requiring again
higher external 9-ODA levels for suppression. Workers using this pathway are
repelled by higher 9-ODA levels and the external 9-ODA levels perceived by the
worker are reduced.

Laying workers of these dominant subfamilies suppress the ovary activation of other workers by the above described reaction–diffusion mechanism (for a recent review see Neumann and Moritz, 2002). The genotypic structure of the colony thus functions as a facilitator of the self-organisation process as a consequence of a genetically preset individual threshold variability.

Pattern in the colony

Based on these hypotheses which are derived from laboratory experiments, a series of predictions for the spatial arrangement of reproductive workers in the colony emerges. The queen is clearly the main source of queen pheromones in the queenright colony. Usually she patrols the colony thereby spreading her pheromones. Although the spread of her pheromones is enhanced further by 'messenger' workers (Velthuis, 1972; Seeley, 1979), one would expect a diffusion gradient around her with the area near the queen having a higher pheromone concentration than areas far away from the queen. If so, workers distant from the queen would be expected to develop a more queen-like mandibular gland secretion than those in close proximity to the queen. This was tested by confining the queen to a specific location on the comb. Through this experimental intervention there were workers that were rarely in contact with the queen and other workers that were often in very close contact. Indeed, workers distant from the queen developed a much more queen-like mandibular gland secretion than workers that were in close proximity to the queen (Moritz et al., 2001). In a similar subsequent experiment in three queenless colonies, workers with a high queen/worker substance ratio in their mandibular gland secretions met less frequently with workers that had a more queen-like ratio (Fig. 3.3). Subordinate workers with a low production of queen substance were more often attracted to dominant workers. This further corroborated the above notion that the pheromonal blend released by the mandibular glands is a good candidate to serve as a central cue in the regulation of reproductive dominance in honeybee workers. Since there was strong genetic variance for attraction or repellence to pseudoqueens and real queens (Moritz et al., 2001) it seems that genetically determined initial minute threshold differences among workers are amplified by negative feedback loops finally yielding the extreme phenotypes.

Task specialisation

Genotypic variance is an important factor for division of labour in honeybee colonies, because the list of genetically determined specialist tasks for individual workers is long. They include foraging (nectar, pollen and water:

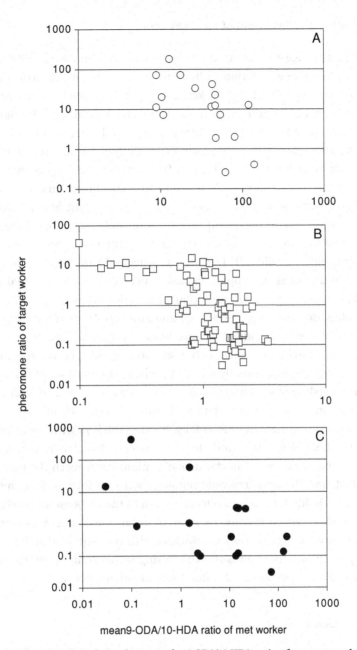

Figure 3.3 Correlation between the 9-ODA/10-HDA ratio of a target worker with workers that she met in a five-day observation period. Freshly emerged workers ($n = 16(A), 108(B), 17(C)$, respectively) were individually labelled and observed in three observation colonies (A, B, C). Over a period of five days the position of the workers was monitored in six daily observations scans. Two workers 'met' if they were observed at the same location on the comb. In all three colonies workers with high 9-ODA levels 'met' on the average more often with workers that had a low 9-ODA/10-HDA ratio at the end of the observation period. Thus pheromonally 'dominant' workers avoided each other but attracted subordinate ones. The overall intracolonial Spearman's rank correlation is $r_S = -0.23750$ ($n = 107$; $p = 0.014$).

Kryger *et al.*, 2000; Page *et al.*, 2000), defensive behaviour (Hunt *et al.*, 1999), reproduction and pheromone secretion (Hillesheim *et al.*, 1989) among many others. But this does not mean that these workers carry 'specialist' alleles at specific loci that invariably enable them to perform the tasks they specialise in. Though this has been shown to be true for pollen foraging in great detail (Hunt *et al.*, 1995a, b; Page *et al.*, 2000), and may be true for various other traits, it seems to be a rather extreme assumption for the general functioning of task specialisation in honeybee colonies. If only specific alleles allow workers to perform certain tasks, this would frequently result in colonies that by chance might have no workers at all that specialise in an important task if these alleles were rare. Unless the queen would be able to select males carrying complementing specific specialist alleles, most colonies would fail. This seems rather unlikely because the queen mates in flight and does not appear to have much control over the males she mates with. A more likely scenario is that of genetic variance for behavioural thresholds (Robinson and Page, 1988; Page and Mitchell, 1998). If a certain environmental cue exceeds an individual threshold, the specific behaviour will be released in that individual. Under such a scenario genetic specialists will also develop but it will depend strongly on the genotypic composition of the colony rather than on task specific genotypes (Fig. 3.4). A worker bee that specialised in nectar foraging in one colony (e.g. from subfamily 4 in Fig. 3.4A) might not have become a nectar forager in another colony. If other workers with lower release thresholds for this task (e.g. subfamily 10 in Fig. 3.4B) switched to nectar foraging much sooner, the intracolonial nectar demand might never reach the threshold of subfamily 4, and the workers would not engage in this form of foraging. The same argument holds for our case where we study the response of workers to queen pheromone concentrations. As soon as intracolonial queen pheromone levels drop below a certain threshold, workers with the highest threshold start producing pheromone themselves thereby raising intracolonial pheromone levels and keeping them above the threshold for the other workers.

Conclusion

Reproduction of workers is an important aspect of the life history of the honeybee (Moritz *et al.*, 1998). The queen pheromones are a central signal in establishing worker reproductive hierarchies, but when the queen is lost, workers may use them too. The loss of the queen results in a predictable pattern of laying activity of workers. The few workers that develop into pseudoqueens are selected after a severe intracolonial competition. Based on their individual inhibition threshold and the propensity to be attracted or repelled by queen pheromones, a reaction–diffusion-like mechanism as described in Fig. 3.2 can explain the

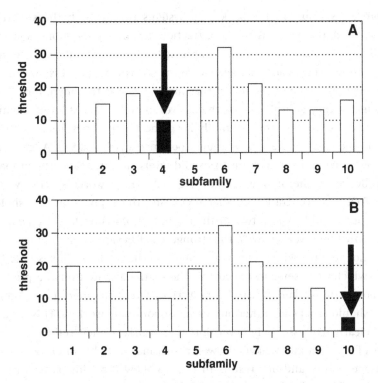

Figure 3.4 The queen most probably has no means to select her mating partner on the basis of their quality in producing an efficient mix of matching genetic specialists in the colony. Workers of a given patriline with the lowest threshold (arrows) specialise in a given task (e.g. nectar foraging) depending on their individual threshold and the patriline composition of the colony. Whereas workers of patriline 4 have the lowest threshold in colony A (top) and would be the first to be involved in nectar foraging, they would not in colony B (bottom). Worker specialisation thus depends on the colony composition and is expected to be determined by chance to a great extent, unless there are very strong gene effects (see text for an example on pollen foraging).

development of worker reproduction. In such a model the *reaction* of the worker is the change of the individual suppression threshold to the queen substance concentration, which forms a cloud around the pheromone source. The workers change their own 9-ODA production thereby changing the local 9-ODA levels in the colony. The locally perceived pheromone concentration may cause two effects:

(1) it enhances attraction or repellence to the pheromone source
(2) it changes the suppression threshold level of the individual worker.

Both processes result in feedback loop systems tuning both the suppression threshold and the propensity for attraction towards pheromone sources by the worker (Fig. 3.2). As a result, suppressed workers are attracted to strong pheromone sources, which further reduce the individual suppression threshold. This in turn raises the attraction of the worker towards the pheromone source. Consequently, they actively expose themselves to higher 9-ODA levels. Dominant workers avoid sources of royal mandibular gland pheromones. Because they are distant to the pheromone source, they experience a reduced 9-ODA level, which raises the individual suppression threshold levels, and increases the propensity for repellence to pheromone sources (Fig. 3.2). These workers actively search for low 9-ODA concentration further increasing the suppression threshold. As a result one would expect two distinct types of workers: few pseudoqueens, because only those workers with the strongest 9-ODA signals and highest thresholds are not suppressed by others, and many sterile workers. This is exactly the pattern, which we observe in the colony. The spatial distribution of reproductive and subordinate workers must also be very different in the colony. Dominant workers should repel each other but attract subordinate workers. This behaviour is most clearly expressed whenever dominant workers elicit retinue behaviour in a set of subordinate workers. However, this may only be an extreme case of pheromone action, and our results in Fig. 3.3 show that this pattern can also be observed in the colony without actual retinues. Small dynamic pheromone fluctuations may therefore govern the establishment of reproductive hierarchies.

Polyandry, resulting in an unpredictable mix of genotypes in the colony, is nevertheless the base structure for establishing genetic reproductive hierarchies among the workers. We suggest that the genetically determined minute differences in individual threshold responses are enhanced by subsequent self-organised mechanisms. The final phenotype is thus not the direct effect of a specific gene for a certain trait, but rather the result of worker–worker interactions that are controlled by at least two feedback loops (Fig. 3.2). The gene does not determine alone whether or not a specific worker develops into a pseudoqueen. The presence of a 'dominance' allele (e.g. for a high threshold or queen repellence) may enhance the probability of a worker becoming a pseudoqueen. In the end, however, the realised reproductive hierarchies will entirely depend on the other workers and the subfamily composition of the colony.

In light of the novel developments of pheromone trapping from live honeybee workers (Crewe et al., 2004), the methodological basis seems to be set to tackle the proximate mechanisms of this phenomenon in even further detail. Advanced genomics may provide an understanding of the regulation of the actual genes involved that set the initial threshold differences. The future for understanding the organisation of insect colonies such as those of honeybees will lie in a combined approach including system theory, genetics, sociobiology and biochemistry.

Acknowledgements

We thank the Deutsche Forschungsgemeinschaft and the National Research Foundation for financial support. Part of this research was facilitated through an Alexander von Humboldt Senior Research Award (NRF) to RFAM.

References

Alber, M., Jordan, R., Ruttner, F. and Ruttner, H. (1955). Von der Paarung der Honigbiene. *Z. Bienenforsch.* **3**, 1–28.

Boomsma, J. J. and Ratnieks, F. L. W. (1996). Paternity in eusocial Hymenoptera. *Phil. Trans. Roy. Soc. London B* **351**, 947–975.

Butler, C. G. (1959). Queen substance. *Bee World* **40**, 269–275.

Butler, C. G., Callow, R. K., Johnston, F. R. S. and Johnston, N. C. (1962). The isolation and synthesis of queen substance, 9-oxodec-*trans*-2-enoic acid, a honeybee pheromone. *Proc. Roy. Entomol. Soc. London* **155**, 417–432.

Crewe, R. M., Moritz, R. F. A. and Lattorff, M. (2004). Using silicon tubes for trapping volatile compounds on biological surfaces *in vivo*. *Chemoecol.* **14**, 77–79.

Crozier, R. H. and Fjerdingstad, E. J. (2001). Polyandry in social Hymenoptera: disunity in diversity? *Ann. Zool. Fenn.* **38**, 267–285.

Haberl, M. and Tautz, D. (1998). Sperm usage in honey bees. *Behav. Ecol. Sociobiol.* **42**, 247–255.

Hamilton, W. D. (1964a). The genetical evolution of social behaviour. I. *J. Theoret. Biol.* **7**, 1–16.

(1964b). The genetical evolution of social behaviour. II. *J. Theoret. Biol.* **7**, 17–52.

Hillesheim, E., Koeniger, N. and Moritz, R. F. A. (1989). Colony performance in honeybees (*Apis mellifera capensis*) depends on the proportion of subordinate and dominant workers. *Behav. Ecol. Sociobiol.* **24**, 291–296.

Hunt, G. J., Page, R. E. and Fondrk, M. K. (1995a). Identification of quantitative trait loci that affect pollen-hoarding behavior in the honeybee. *J. Cell Biochem.* Suppl. **21A**, 196–198.

(1995b). Major quantitative trait loci affecting honeybee foraging behavior. *Genetics* **141**, 1537–1545.

Hunt, G. J., Collins, A. M, Rivera, R., Page, R. E. and Guzman-Novoa, E. (1999). Quantitative trait loci influencing honeybee alarm pheromone levels. *J. Hered.* **90**, 585–589.

Kryger, P., Kryger, U. and Moritz, R. F. A. (2000). Genotypical variability for the tasks of water collecting and scenting in a honey bee colony. *Ethology* **106**, 769–779.

Moritz, R. F. A. and Hillesheim, E. (1985). Inheritance of dominance in honeybees (*Apis mellifera capensis*). *Behav. Ecol. Sociobiol.* **17**, 87–89.

Moritz, R. F. A., Kryger, P. and Koeniger, G. *et al.* (1995). High degree of polyandry in *Apis dorsata* queens detected by microsatellite variability. *Behav. Ecol. Sociobiol.* **37**, 357–363.

Moritz, R. F. A., Kryger, P. and Allsopp, M. (1996). Competition for royalty in bees. *Nature* **384**, 31.

Moritz, R. F. A., Beye, M. and Hepburn, H. R. (1998). Estimating the contribution of laying workers to population fitness in African honeybees (*Apis mellifera*) with molecular markers. *Insects Soc.* **45**, 277–287.

Moritz, R. F. A., Simon, U. E. and Crewe, R. M. (2000). Pheromonal contest between honeybee workers. *Naturwiss.* **87**, 395–397.

Moritz, R. F. A., Crewe, R. M. and Hepburn, H. R. (2001). The role of the queen in the distribution of workers in the honeybee colony. *Ethology* **107**, 1–13.

Moritz, R. F. A., Crewe, R. M. and Lattorf, M. (2003). Honeybee workers (*Apis mellifera capensis*) compete for producing queen-like pheromone signals. *Proc. Roy. Soc. London* **271**: S98–S100.

Neumann, P. and Moritz, R. F. A. (2002). The Cape Honeybee phenomenon: the sympatric evolution of a social parasite in real time. *Behav. Ecol. Sociobiol.* **52**, 271–281.

Page, R. E. (1986). Sperm utilization in social insects. *Annu. Rev. Entomol.* **10**, 359–361.

Page, R. E. and Mitchell, S. D. (1998). Self-organization and the evolution of division of labor. *Apidologie* **29**, 171–190.

Page, R. E., Fondrk, M. K., Hunt, G. J. *et al.* (2000). Genetic dissection of honeybee (*Apis mellifera* L.) foraging behavior. *J. Hered.* **91**, 474–479.

Palmer, K. and Oldroyd, B. P. (2000). Evolution of multiple mating in the genus *Apis*. *Apidologie* **31**, 235–248.

(2001). Mating frequency in *Apis florea* revisited (Hymenoptera, Apidae). *Insectes Soc.* **48**, 40–43.

Plettner, E., Slessor, K. N., Winston, M. L. and Oliver, J. E. (1996). Caste-selective pheromone biosynthesis in honeybees. *Science* **271**, 1851–1853.

Plettner, E., Slessor, K. N. and Winston, M. L. (1998). Biosynthesis of mandibular acids in honey bees (*Apis mellifera*): *de novo* synthesis, route of fatty acid hydroxylation and caste selective beta-oxidation. *Insect Biochem. Mol. Biol.* **28**, 31–42.

Ratnieks, F. L. W. (1988). Reproductive harmony via mutual policing by workers in eusocial insects. *Am. Naturalist* **132**, 217–236.

Robinson, G. E. and Page, R. E. (1988). Genetic determination of guarding and undertaking in honey bee colonies. *Nature* **333**, 356–358.

Schlüns, H., Moritz, R. F. A. and Kryger, P. (2001). Behavioral control over mating frequency in queen honeybees (*Apis mellifera* L.): revisiting the sperm-limitation-hypothesis. In *Proc. 2001 Berlin Mg European Sections of IUSSI*, p. 105.

Seeley, T. D. (1979). Queen substance dispersal by messenger workers in honeybee colonies. *Behav. Ecol. Sociobiol.* **5**, 391–415.

Simon, U. E., Moritz, R. F. A. and Crewe, R. M. (2001). The ontogenetic pattern of mandibular gland components in queenless worker bees (*Apis mellifera capensis* Esch.). *J. Insect Physiol.* **47**, 735–738.

Strassmann, J. (2001). The rarity of multiple mating by females in the social Hymenoptera. *Insectes Soc.* **48**, 1–13.

Taber, S. (1955). Sperm distribution in the spermathecae of multiple-mated queen honey bees. *J. Econ. Entomol.* **48**, 522–525.

Tarpy, D. R. and Page, R. E. (2000). No behavioral control over mating frequency in queen honeybees (*Apis mellifera* L.): implications for the evolution of extreme polyandry. *Am. Naturalist* **155**, 820–827.

Turing, A. (1952). The chemical basis of morphogenesis. *Phil. Trans. Roy. Soc. London B* **237**, 37–72.

Velthuis, H. H. W. (1972). Observations of the transmission of queen substances in the honeybee colony by the attendants of the queen. *Behaviour* **41**, 105–129.

Winston, M. L. and Slessor, K. N. (1992). The essence of royalty: honey bee queen pheromone. *Am. Sci.* **80**, 374–385.

(1998). Honey bee primer pheromones and colony organization: gaps in our knowledge. *Apidologie* **29**, 81–95.

Wossler, T. C. (2002). Pheromone mimicry by *Apis mellifera capensis* social parasites leads to reproductive anarchy in host *Apis mellifera scutellata* colonies. *Apidologie* **33**, 139–163.

Woyke, J. (1960). Natural and artificial insemination of queen honey bees. *Pszczelnicze Zeszyty Naukowe* **4**, 183–275.

4

Traffic rules of fish schools: a review of agent-based approaches

JULIA K. PARRISH
University of Washington

STEVEN V. VISCIDO
Northwest Fisheries Science Center, Seattle

Introduction

Perhaps no other group of organisms typifies emergent pattern as a function of the collective as well as schools of fish. Ranging in numbers from tens to millions, across all aquatic environments, trophic levels, and phylogenetic groups, fish schools are a quintessential biological model of collective action because: (1) the range of group pattern and behaviour appears to retain fundamental similarities across taxa, suggesting underlying mechanism, and (2) individuals are clearly not related to each other, as are social insects, and therefore pattern can not be simply explained by kinship altruism. Thus, schooling remains both a fundamental biological phenomenon, and a mystery. This chapter explores agent-based approaches to the study of fish schooling, with an eye towards synthesizing approaches and findings to date, and examining the degree to which synthetic results match data collected from real schools.

Specifically we will: (1) discuss emergence versus epiphenomena in the context of the individual, the group and the population; (2) review the major agent-based approaches to the study of fish schooling, with an in-depth examination of the 'traffic rules of fish schools'; (3) compare simulation and model output to positional data collected on fish in real schools; and (4) suggest future directions for the study of fish schooling.

Self-Organisation and Evolution of Social Systems, ed. Charlotte K. Hemelrijk.
Published by Cambridge University Press. © Cambridge University Press 2005.

Emergence versus epiphenomena

We begin with a caveat: the majority of studies on fish schooling to date have centred on the question of why fish school, that is, the proximate and ultimate mechanisms behind the evolution of schooling behaviour (Pitcher and Parrish 1993). Within the last two decades this work has evolved into a detailed examination of the moment-to-moment choices individual fish make, a cost–benefit (i.e. economic) approach to grouping behaviour in fish (e.g. Nonacs *et al.*, 1998; Krause and Ruxton, 2002). Here, the essential question is whether membership in a group is beneficial to the individual; if so, under what circumstances; and who 'pays' the cost of an individual's benefit (Hamner and Parrish, 1997)? We will not explicitly delve into this literature, but instead address the sister question: *how* do fish school? How are groups formed and maintained given limited sensory and cognitive abilities of the individual members? These questions require an examination of the physical and physiological limitations of the system, and ultimately of the processing capabilities of the agents. Thus, although forcing factors selecting for gregariousness are not explored, the underlying assumption in this approach is that grouping is adaptive.

Early work, both scientific and literary (e.g. Steinbeck and Ricketts, 1941), described schools as super-organisms where individual fish acted collectively, apparently guided by an unseen hand. Schools display an impressive array of group-level phenomena, including even density profiles, polarity, distinct edges, distinct shape, and coordinated movement. Our current understanding of these group-level patterns emerging from the local interactions between neighbours (as opposed to direction from a higher power or as a result of omniscient individuals) is the result of the development of evolutionary biology and specifically of the model of the individual as selfish (e.g. Williams, 1966; Wilson, 1975). Although the individual-based nature of fish schooling is now taken as a given, what remains unclear is the degree to which observed pattern is in itself the product of ensuing selection, or merely a by-product of self-organisation (e.g. epiphenomena: Levin, 1999; Camazine *et al.*, 2001). We refer to the interaction between self-organisation and ensuing selection as emergence.

It is tempting to postulate that all attributes of a school have definitive fitness functions enabling in the simplest sense members to increase their fitness over non-members, and coordinated groups to have a higher average fitness relative to uncoordinated ones. Perhaps there were some number of group-level patterns that were selected against, because groups displaying them attracted more predators or dispersed food more quickly, leaving members proximately with lower body condition and ultimately with lower reproduction and survival capabilities (Bakun and Cury, 1999; Parrish and Edelstein-Keshet, 2000). Although individual schools do not enjoy selective advantage, as membership is a fluid process among schools, schools within an oceanic region may have enjoyed selective advantage (Bakun and Cury, 1999). However, inanimate particles can display many of the same visual patterns as are seen in animate aggregations (Vicsek *et al.*, 1995), arguing for observed pattern as epiphenomena (Levin, 1999) without selective advantage. In fact, it is possible that observed pattern may even be disadvantageous to individual members, owing to factors such as predator attraction to large masses of prey (Parrish, 1992). The relationship between emergent pattern versus epiphenomena, self-organisation versus selective forcing, and individual versus group selection has yet to be comprehensively explored in either modelling or experimental work.

Why should biologists study self-organisation? Fundamentally we study self-organisation because it is fascinating to a human to watch 'simple' animals doing things like wheeling together in unison without any obvious cues. Fish schools and bird flocks are doing something even humans can't do unless, for example, they drill for a long time with an expert marching band instructor. This makes us curious about what is going on, and how it came to be. On a scientific level, can agent-based approaches facilitate an ecological or evolutionary approach to the study of gregarious behaviour? Can simulating how fish school address why fish school? Agent-based approaches – using only local rules – are powerful because they are constraining. That is, rather than simply taking an optimality approach (i.e., joining a group is beneficial) agent-based approaches allow the detailed study of exactly how an organism can aggregate and where it will be in the group. Thus, we can also study what individuals are prevented from doing. For instance, when predators threaten, optimality models suggest individuals should move to the centre; however, the actual movement of individuals is constrained by the arrangement and movement patterns of neighbours preventing simple unconstrained locomotion on the part of any individual (Parrish, 1989). Ultimately, we believe it is a combination of the evolutionary and optimality approaches with the more detailed agent-based study of self-organisation that will truly explain the persistent existence of emergent group phenomena such as schooling.

Agent-based approaches to fish schooling

Biological beginnings

Two classic papers provided an early foundation for agent-based modelling of fish schooling behaviour. In 1971, Hamilton published his seminal work, 'Geometry for the selfish herd', which laid out a theoretical basis for predation pressure as the driving mechanism responsible for the maintenance, and perhaps evolution, of gregarious behaviour. In this early model, locally acting agents, knowing only their nearest-neighbour distances and the distances between sets of immediately adjacent neighbours move to insert themselves between neighbours with the smallest inter-individual space. We conceptually reproduce Hamilton's (1971) model as a set of seven nearshore minnows (rather than the original frogs) under the threat of attack by a larger, open-water fish, such as a pike. At each time step, the minnow with the greatest total distance, or gap, between neighbours inserts itself between the nearest possible set of adjacent neighbours with the goal of reducing its domain of danger. Given some minimum limit of nearest-neighbour distance, a single group is quickly formed (Fig. 4.1). Hamilton's (1971) paper spawned a tremendous focus on predation as a mechanism behind the evolution of gregarious behaviour, although debate continues as to whether the model, or its assumptions, are correct (Parrish, 1989; James *et al.*, 2004). Significantly, the model did incorporate both approaches (why and how), an integration which has been largely absent in ensuing work.

In 1976, Breder published 'Fish schools as operational structures', in which he defined a school as 'a closely packed group of very similar individuals united by their uniformity of orientation' and went on to theoretically explore three-dimensional packing arrangements (what became known as the crystalline lattice model: Fig. 4.2) that typify schools. Although this and other early references (e.g. Parr, 1927; Breder, 1951; Van Olst and Hunter, 1970; Shaw, 1978) did not explicitly describe agent-based approaches, they set the stage for the study of emergent properties by attempting to describe the inherent pattern in schooling, including regularity and architecture of packing, polarity, group shape and activity synchronization. In this sense, and especially in the case of Breder (1976), the stage was set for future simulations that would attempt to mimic these group-level phenomena. However (and not least of which because actual measurements were, and are, tremendously difficult to obtain), data on the behaviour of fish moving in actual schools was, and is, largely lacking. Thus, what we think is happening, rather than what is actually happening, partially formed the foundation of research into fish school self-organisation, and this continues to be the case today.

Chronological review of agent-based models

Agent-based approaches to simulating fish schooling have generally adopted a 'sum-of-forces' approach, with varying numbers and functional forms of forces, depending on the model. Forces are applied according to zones of interaction (Fig. 4.3), most commonly repulsion, alignment, attraction and search, as

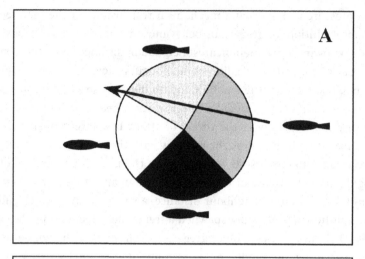

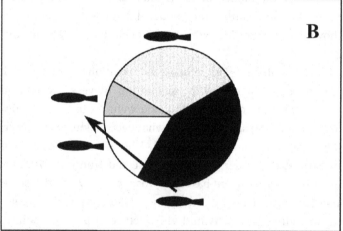

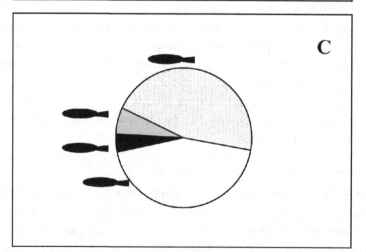

Figure 4.1

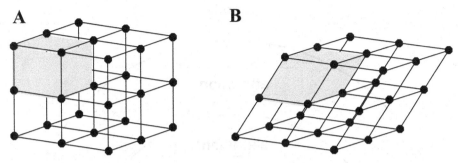

Figure 4.2 Spatial lattices in perspective view showing (A) a cubic lattice, and (B) a rhomboidal lattice. A single cell of each is shown as solid. If each lattice point is taken to be the centroid of a single fish, and if all individuals are aligned, then the lattice structures superficially resemble fish schools. Redrawn from Figure 1 in Breder (1976).

a function of distance from the agent of interest. In the aggregate, forces dictate either resultant direction or velocity. Additional forces, applied without reference to distance between agents, may include a random component of movement, a directed component of movement, and frictional drag. Finally, some models adopt a predetermined speed (i.e. fixed or randomly chosen from a normal distribution) to simplify the calculations. Most models have been restricted to two dimensions, a relatively small number of fish (2–20) and reduction to points (that is, the agents do not possess mass or volume).

Early work was concerned with the basic question: under what conditions will groups form and persist? Breder (1954) suggested an attraction and repulsion approach, where the former force was uniformly applied and the latter force declined as the square of the distance between adjacent fish. Perhaps because this early paper did not include a simulation per se, it seems to have quickly vanished from view once true sum-of-forces simulations began to appear. Inagaki *et al.* (1976) formulated an early sum-of-forces simulation with three forces: social force (zoned-based attraction and repulsion), swimming force (a set speed imposed on the agents) and random force. Agents averaged the influence

Figure 4.1 (*cont.*) A depiction of the original 'selfish herd' model by Hamilton (1971). Shaded regions represent the Domains of Danger (DOD) for each fish. (A) In the initial starting position, the fish with the grey region finds the smaller of the two adjacent gaps. (B) After moving into the small gap, the fish with the grey region has reduced his DOD, at the expense of his neighbours. The fish with the black region now has the largest DOD, and thus moves into the smaller of the two adjacent gaps. (C) Final positions for all four fish, with the grey and black regions indicating that the 'selfish' fish have drastically reduced their Domains of Danger.

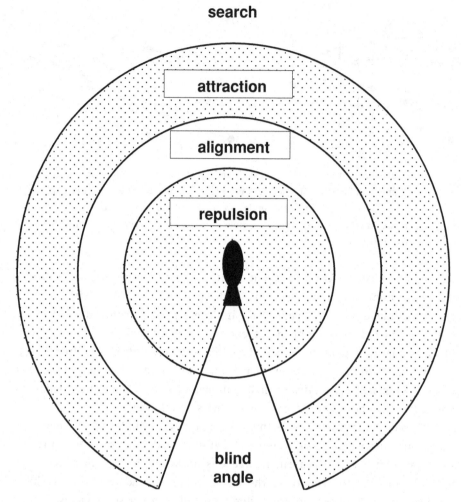

Figure 4.3 Schematic representing a typical 'zone-based' model, showing zones of search, attraction, alignment and repulsion, as well as the 'blind angle' behind the fish where it cannot see any neighbours.

of all other agents within the social force zones. Cursory examination of the parameter space indicated that inclusion of social force was necessary to produce cohesion, whereas inclusion of swimming and random forces balanced the tendency for individuals to form a dense, static group. Sakai (1973, as reported in Niwa, 1994) also produced an early sum-of-forces simulation indicating that group structure and motion were dependent on inclusion of both attraction and alignment. These early papers both suggested that a balance of forces is necessary for the formation of groups with flexible membership and the ability to traverse space.

Aoki (1982, 1984) extended these results with a more comprehensive sum-of-forces model including zone-based repulsion, alignment, attraction and random search, with velocity derived from a set distribution. The relative influence of neighbours was distance-based, included a blind zone of 30 degrees, and was limited to four individuals, even if the school was larger. Output was reported as net *individual* displacement, and compactness of the *group*, starting an important trend in reporting metrics at individual, group, and/or population levels (Parrish *et al.*, 2002). Aoki's models represent a conceptual difference from earlier models, shifting the emphasis from grouping per se to a concentration on the cohesive movement of the group. In other words, given the group exists, under what conditions will it react as a whole? Removing the attraction/repulsion force caused agents to disperse, whereas removing alignment caused the group to wheel (decreased net displacement). Thus, Aoki concluded that both attraction and alignment were necessary to form groups and maintain group cohesion, respectively; and these papers were the progenitors of the series of simulations that included alignment as a default parameter.

In the early 1990s, simulations of fish schooling began to blossom. Most authors based their simulations on the earlier work, especially of Aoki (1982, 1984), extending the sum-of-forces approach to consider what happened to group cohesion as the number of influential neighbours or the weighting of those neighbours changed, the size of zones (e.g. Fig. 4.3) changed, or the functional form of the social forces (attraction and repulsion) were altered. Warburton and Lazarus (1991) constructed a simple two-dimensional model that systematically explored the functional relationship between social force and group cohesion. Here, the integrated forces of attraction and repulsion were modelled as linear, exponential or asymptotic, where the latter two functions encompassed a family of formulae. School sizes were small (two to nine) and agents considered all neighbours. Linear and positively asymptotic functions yielded not only cohesive groups (measured as mean inter-individual distance) but stable ones (measured as coefficient of variation in inter-individual distance); all other functions lead to similarly cohesive but unstable groups (i.e. high coefficient of variation) or less cohesive (i.e. high inter-individual distance) and unstable groups. Within a functional form, increasing the group size increased both cohesion and stability. That paper set the stage for further exploration of the issue of stability, and was in this sense a precursor to the use of fitness algorithms linked to stable expression of group pattern (e.g. Hiramatsu *et al.*, 2000).

In a model nearly identical to that of Aoki (1982, 1984), Huth and Wissel (1990) concluded that averaging neighbour influences produced more realistic schooling whereas adopting a priority-weighted choice of influential neighbours (the decision model) produced 'confusion'. These results were extended two years later (Huth and Wissel, 1992) to examine the impact of altering zone size. Not surprisingly, they found that changing the size of the alignment zone (from 0 to 10 body lengths) had the greatest effect on both polarity and expanse, whereas altering the zone of repulsion (0–3 body lengths) or attraction (0–6 body lengths) had minor to inconsequential effects. In 1994, these same authors extended their earlier simulations to three dimensions, with no change in major conclusions (Huth and Wissel, 1994).

Huth and Wissel (1990, 1992, 1994) introduced two important, and perhaps subtle, changes to agent-based models of fish schooling. First, there is an element of circularity in their approach. Unlike their group-level output expanse, polarity was specifically pre-programmed to exist as the zone-based alignment force. Second, individuals were essentially prevented from leaving the group, as agents farther than the maximum attraction zone distance oriented on their nearest neighbour, and swam directly back to that neighbour (Huth and Wissel, 1992). Thus, the emphasis of these simulations became ever more focused on self-organised pattern within the group rather than on the existence of groups, to the point where fission was prevented and the group became synonymous with the population.

During the same period, Reuter and Breckling (1994) published a simulation similar to that of Huth and Wissel (1992) and Aoki (1982), with a few crucial differences: upper limits of school size were dramatically larger (50 as opposed to 8); individuals reacted to a distance-based weighted average ($1/D$ or $1/D^2$) of *all* neighbours (rather than just four); and the size of the attraction zone was extended greatly (from 5 body lengths described in Aoki (1982) and Huth and Wissel (1992) to 17 body lengths). The latter two conditions preclude stragglers, and are effectively identical to the directed search condition of Huth and Wissel (1992). One interesting innovation in this model was an exploration of the percentage of time fish could act differently (modelled as only repulsion functioning) and still remain aggregated (Fig. 4.4). Beneath a threshold of 40–50% of the time-steps acting individually did not change group characteristics. This result presaged both an exploration of individuality (e.g. Romey, 1996) and group memory resident in the arrangement of individuals (e.g. Couzin *et al.*, 2002).

Although schooling behaviour (measured as high polarity and low nearest-neighbour distance) was produced, the Reuter and Breckling (1994) paper raised the interesting question of how many neighbours a fish can actually sense and incorporate into decision-making, as well as the functional shape of that integration. That is, can a fish sense the velocity and acceleration of 49 neighbours? If so, does a fish utilise all of this information in resolving its own movement vector? What is the relative weighting of neighbours? And finally, does that weighting change with circumstances?

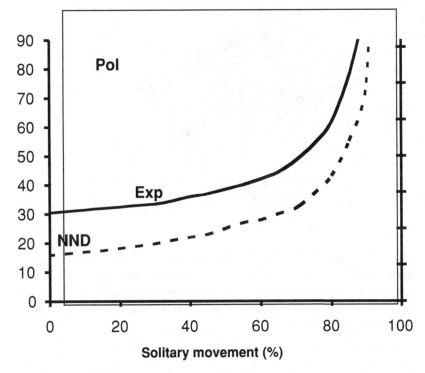

Figure 4.4 The effect of increasing the amount of 'solitary' behaviour on three schooling metrics: polarity (Pol), nearest-neighbour distance (NND) and expanse (Exp). Polarity is rescaled so that a right angle (90°) = 0.0, and perfect alignment (0°) = 0.0. Expanse is the mean distance from each individual in the group to the group's centre. Redrawn from Reuter and Breckling (1994).

Romey (1996) combined the approaches and issues raised by Warburton and Lazarus (1991) and Reuter and Breckling (1994) to create a schooling simulation in which a small number (2–10) of truly omniscient fish (an interaction radius of 100 body lengths) interact with their neighbours. Each fish behaved according to different distance-weighted social force functions – in other words, simulated fish had permanent individuality. Although both pure and mixed strategy groups remained aggregated, there were three very interesting results at the individual and group levels, respectively. First, individuals within the group sorted by strategy, a by-product of the fact that differing attraction/repulsion functions result in different equilibrium distances (preferred near-neighbour distance). Second, even one agent with a different social force function could substantively influence the movement patterns of the group, and that individual did not have to be on the periphery. In other words, leaders can be individuals that react differently (Couzin and Krause, 2003). Third, groups could change from schooling (high net

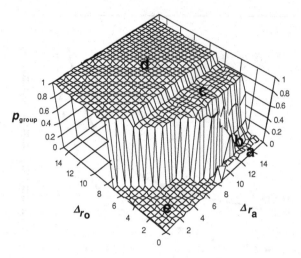

Figure 4.5 Group polarity (p_{group}) as a function of the size of the attraction (Δr_a) and orientation (Δr_o) zones. Here, $p_{\text{group}} = 1$ represents perfect alignment, and $p_{\text{group}} = 0$ represents disarray. Lower-case letters represent (a) swarm, (b) torus, (c) dynamically parallel and (d) highly polarised groups. From Couzin *et al.* (2002); reprinted with permission.

displacement, low turning rate) to milling (vice versa) by altering group size, even within some pure social force groups. Subsequent agent-based simulations have confirmed sorting by strategy (ungulates: Gueron *et al.*, 1996; fish: Couzin *et al.*, 2002; primates: Hemelrijk, 2000; traffic: Helbing and Huberman, 1998) and leader effects (Gueron *et al.*, 1996).

Couzin *et al.* (2002) greatly extended the work of earlier authors by exploring the relative zone size of the three social forces (repulsion, alignment, attraction) and the degree of individuality (modelled as an error term in resultant direction *sensu* Viscek *et al.* (1995)) in a three-dimensional simulation of up to 100 agents. Output variables included polarity, angular momentum and group shape/activity. This paper significantly advanced agent-based approaches applied to fish schools because it truly explored resultant group pattern over a range of input parameter space (Fig. 4.5). Not surprisingly, the size of the alignment zone (termed orientation) largely dictated polarity. What is truly interesting is that transitions between schooling states (fragmented, swarm, torus, dynamically polarised, rigidly polarised) were abrupt, a pattern also described for automobile traffic (Helbing and Huberman, 1998). Discontinuous transition between polarised and unpolarised states had been modelled dynamically by Niwa (1994), who showed that the phase shift depended on the strength of the noise in the system relative to an arrayal (velocity-matching) force. A second noteworthy result from the Couzin *et al.* (2002) simulation was the finding of hysteresis: that both the current parameter states of individuals as well as the architecture dictated by their previous parameter states were important in determining school configuration (Fig. 4.6). Thus, the group possesses a structural memory. This raises questions about the degree to which current shape, size or activity dictates the ease, or even availability, of future group-level response.

In contrast to earlier work that adopted the assumption that agent movement was more important than agent substance, Kunz and Hemelrijk (2003) and Viscido *et al.* (2005) chose to impart substance to their agents. Although this is more computationally intensive, there are interesting implications. For instance, Kunz and Hemelrijk (2003) found that agent shape (point, line, ellipse) had a significant effect on several group-level output variables, including polarity (referred to as confusion, or the inverse of polarity), the ratio of first to second nearest-neighbour distances (referred to as homogeneity), group velocity, and group shape (major to minor axis ratio). Obviously, but importantly, differences were ascribed to the altered shape of repulsion, alignment and attraction zones as the agents took on more realistic configurations. Thus large schools of elliptical agents were more densely packed, less polarised, slower and more closely approximating a circle. Our own work (Parrish *et al.*, 2002; Viscido *et al.*, 2005) has imparted both an ellipsoidal shape (three dimensions) and a mass to the agents, and suggests individuals will crash when repulsion functions are too shallow, essentially preventing fish from slowing down fast enough (Viscido *et al.*, unpubl. data).

Hiramatsu *et al.* (2000) extended agent-based schooling simulations by linking the former to a simple genetic algorithm that was used to select 'optimal rules' allowing the model to most closely approximate values observed in schools of Japanese medaka, *Oryzias latipes*. The simulation itself was not innovative (two-dimensional sum-of-forces, including alignment, and random search outside a 50-body-length envelope, $n = 10$ fish); however, the attempt to allow a rule set to evolve is. The algorithm searched over the width of the repulsion and alignment zones, the blind angle, the number of neighbours to pay attention to, and the prioritisation rules for neighbours (front, side, distance or random choice), with the goal of collectively minimising the error in four individual and group-level metrics: nearest-neighbour distance, polarisation, distance to centre (expanse) and fractal dimension of the group trajectory. Although the model fit was high, the optimal parameters were unrealistic: no blind angle, maximised alignment zone, all neighbours are influential. That is, with a maximised alignment zone and all neighbours taken into consideration, it is not surprising that agent fish were highly polarised and swimming in lock step, even if this is unlikely in nature. In fact, these results point up some of the difficulties of the evolutionary

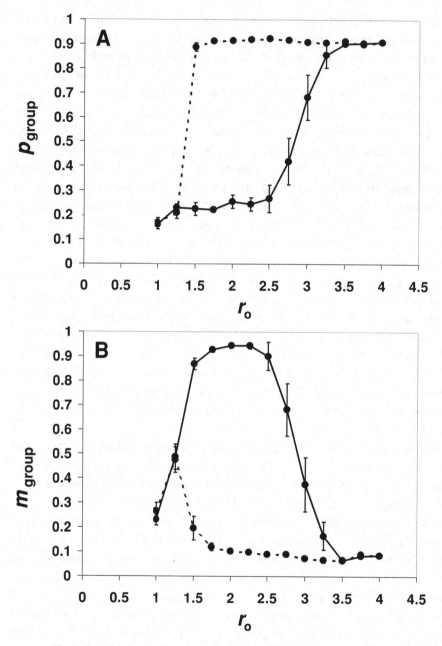

Figure 4.6 Changes in (A) group polarity (p_{group}) and (B) group angular momentum (m_{group}), as individuals within the group decrease (dotted line) or increase (solid line) their zone of orientation (r_o). Group pattern formation depends on the previous history of the group. From Couzin *et al.* (2002); reprinted with permission.

approach. First, an optimal end point must be known. This supposes that we can discern what set of group-level patterns is optimal to the survival of the individual. Second, a choice of rules may obey optimality criteria, but not necessarily embody how real fish school. Finally, at least for the algorithm presented here, optimality is expressed as a total lack of individuality – that is, by minimising error over individual and group-level metrics – even though our inherent understanding of evolution suggests that the ability of individuals to take differential advantage of any situation is ultimately profitable.

Our current simulations are a continuation of the sum-of-forces approach. As with Couzin *et al.* (2002), we have extended into the third dimension and increased the number of agents (to 128). In addition, our agents are physically realistic (they possess a shape and a mass) and have maximum speed and acceleration thresholds observed in real fish of the same size. Finally, our agents are not constrained to constant or predetermined speed, but instead adjust their velocity in response to neighbours. Unlike many previous simulations primarily concerned with emergent pattern within the group, we are also interested in the conditions under which groups form, dissolve and reform. Thus, our zones are not functionally infinite (e.g. Romey, 1996); our fish can become lost.

To understand how emergent properties are affected by population size, we have conducted simulation experiments over populations of 1–128 individuals. We also tested whether emergent properties depended on the number of influential neighbours, by having simulated fish be influenced by 4–24 neighbours as a distance-weighted function. The resulting movement and spatial distributions of our model fish are quantified at the individual, group and population levels using 8–14 metrics averaged over the simulation run (Parrish *et al.*, 2002; Viscido *et al.*, unpubl. data).

Our results showed that group properties such as polarity, group size and group speed are strongly influenced both by population size, and by the number of influential neighbours (Parrish *et al.*, 2002; Viscido *et al.*, unpubl. data). We also found a very strong interaction between the two factors. When individuals responded to all members of the population, groups remained relatively static, milling about in a disorganised fashion. All recorded metrics exhibited anomalies in this area of parameter space (Viscido *et al.*, unpubl. data). Furthermore, as the number of influential neighbours climbed above 16, breakdown in school structure occurred, as individuals unsuccessfully attempted to balance competing influences of too many neighbour positions and velocities (Parrish *et al.*, 2002; Viscido *et al.*, unpubl. data). When the population size far exceeded the number of influential neighbours, each fish took cues from a different, but overlapping, set of neighbours, which resulted in more mobile schools. Because most fish schools are mobile and do not exhibit the static, milling behaviours our simulated fish exhibited when each individual was paying attention to the entire population, we concluded that real fish probably do not pay attention to all other members of the school, even when school size is fairly small. It is also possible to disperse a mill with the addition of an alignment force (e.g. Couzin *et al.*, 2002).

Although studies often use substantially the same forces (attraction, repulsion, alignment, random movement), and generally use the same format (regions, or 'zones', of repulsion, alignment, attraction and random search) (Fig. 4.3), most studies do not systematically vary all factors, and so the relative importance of each factor has remained a mystery (Parrish *et al.*, 2002). To address this important problem, our most recent simulations have explored the degree to which social versus physical forces (or swimming force *sensu* Inagaki *et al.* (1976) and Niwa (1994)) shape school behaviour and structure at the individual, group and population levels, given a constant population size (128 fish) and number of influential neighbours (16).

We have constructed simulations that systematically vary five input parameters (attraction/repulsion, neighbour influence, alignment, drag and random movement), and compared the results against a 'base case' that included a piecewise linear attraction–repulsion function (i.e. with a neutral zone 1 body length wide at $F = 0$), uniform neighbour influence, no alignment force, medium randomness, and no drag. Social forces include attraction–repulsion functional form (linear, curvilinear), alignment force (constant, peaked, decreasing curvilinear) assigned within the neutral zone, and the shape of the distance-weighting function of neighbour influence (decreasing linear, decreasing logistic). Physical, or swimming, forces include drag (drag coefficient of 0.01 or 0.02) and random force (mean of zero with low, medium and high variance). We have computed 11 schooling properties, four at the individual level (path curvature, fractal dimension, nearest-neighbour distance, net-to-gross displacement), four at the group level (group speed, polarity, group size and expanse), and three at the population level (number of groups, number of stragglers collision rate).

For the parameter space we examined, we found that physical forces did not provoke changes in schooling metrics once included in the simulations – that is, the functional forms of random force and drag were inconsequential. However, the actual inclusion of drag did have a large effect (Viscido *et al.*, unpubl. data). This same pattern was also evident for alignment. However, all schooling metrics were highly sensitive to both inclusion and functional form of the remaining social factors: attraction–repulsion and neighbour influence. Changing the attraction–repulsion function caused fish to become denser as the repulsion function became shallower; this resulted in slower-moving groups in which individuals crashed into each other far more frequently than the base case (Viscido *et al.*, unpubl. data). By contrast, discounting neighbour influence as a function of distance rank created small, fast, diffuse groups in which individuals constantly became lost.

Cellular automata models

Although not adopted by the majority of researchers interested in discerning traffic rules for fish schools, cellular automata models have been illustrative vis-à-vis metrics at the group–population boundary (e.g. number of schools, school activity). Here, individual movement is reduced to a set of compass directions based on the symmetry of a two-dimensional grid (e.g. rectangular: Vabø and Nøttestad, 1997; hexagonal: Stöcker, 1999). Fish move at constant velocity (one cell per time-step) to the adjacent cells according to local rules essentially identical to the previously described models. One of the benefits of this approach is the ability to return to the questions examined by Inagaki *et al.* (1976) and others: under what conditions will schools form, and what is the relationship between local rules and school size?

Stöcker (1999) used a cellular automata approach to examine within-school architecture and maximum school size given energetic constraints, including drafting advantages (*sensu* Weihs 1973, 1975) and crowding disadvantages (e.g. oxygen depletion: McFarland and Moss, 1967). Movement rules were constructed according to zone-based repulsion (full cells could not be entered), alignment, attraction and random search, respectively. Output included the number and size of schools, polarisation, and school shape. Not surprisingly, agent alignment was always perfect, a consequence of the rule set and the hexagonal grid. More interesting was the prediction that school size was proportional to a power function of population size, with an exponent of less than 1. Optimality models clearly predict an optimal-to-critical group size independent of population size, that is, based solely on resource limitation (Clark and Mangel, 1984; Duffy and Wissel, 1988). By contrast, agent-based approaches appear to suggest that at restricted local population sizes, group size may be affected by the aggregation rules themselves (e.g. Bonabeau *et al.*, 1999; Stöcker, 1999). Vabø and Nøttestad (1997) used a 900-agent cellular automata model to examine assembly dynamics, school size and school activity with and without predators. Model schools appeared to perform 'classic' predator-avoidance activities, including split, join, vacuole and fountain (Pitcher and Parrish, 1993; Nøttestad and Axelsen, 1999). Fission–fusion rates, and the consequent school size distribution, were dependent on agent, and predator, perception distance (Vabø and Nøttestad, 1997).

Approaches from outside biology

Models of self-organised schools have not only come from the biological literature, but from the physics, systems engineering, artificial life and animation literature as well. Although these papers are much less well cited, if at all, by biologists, there are some very interesting approaches and results. In what has almost become a cult classic, Reynolds (1987) published a qualitative description of a simulation used to ultimately produce an early computer animation *Stella Meets Stanley*, which featured both schooling fish and flocking birds. The simulation was a sum-of-forces with velocity matching of near neighbours. Neighbour influence was forward-weighted and distance-based ($1/D^2$). A separate 'steer-to-avoid' routine allowed agents to negotiate static objects in the environment. Although many current authors cite this paper as a model of the correct approach, it is important to remember what Reynolds was trying to produce: realistic *looking* animal aggregation. In fact, he was not trying to explore the rule space over which actual fish, or birds, might self-organise. This is an important distinction, because it explains the inclusion of terms that are biologically improbable, such as a forward target point to which all agents are attracted (the migratory urge), or agent knowledge of the group centroid within a perception neighbourhood (flock centring).

Sannomiya and colleagues have published a series of papers on schooling fish simulations, based in part on measurements of trajectories of bitterling (*Rhodeus ocellatus ocellatus*) swimming around the edges of a two-dimensionalised (7 cm in depth) tank (Sannomiya and Matuda, 1984; Sannomiya *et al.*, 1990; Doustari and Sannomiya, 1992, 1993a, b, 1995). Later versions of their simulation (Sannomiya and Doustari, 1996), a two-dimensional, sum-of-forces model with repulsion, attraction, and 'characteristic' individual speed ($n = 5$ fish), explored the change in output (school trajectory, lineal size of the school, number of fish in each school) as a function of the number of influential neighbours with respect to individual position, and individual velocity (M_b and M_c, respectively). Although the trajectories were unrealistic (circles and unclosed curves), the model did indicate that changing the number of influential neighbours had dramatic effects on both school size (number of fish) and inter-fish distance. Changing the number of neighbours over which position was assessed had a significant effect on group size, whereas altering the number of neighbours over which velocity was assessed had little effect. Biologically, these results are interesting because they begin to suggest which types of information fish may be gathering from neighbours.

A less-well-known paper published by Viscek *et al.* (1995) examined the state changes in group-to-population level organisation in a two-dimensional system with hundreds to thousands of agents. Agent speed was set, but direction was chosen as an average of all neighbours within an interaction distance. Noise (an added term to resultant direction) and density (either as total number of agents and/or size of the universe) were manipulated. At high densities, no discrete groups formed, but the population moved either coherently in the same direction (low noise) or randomly with some very local correlation (high noise). However, at both low noise and low density, small groups tended to form, where individuals within the groups moved coherently whereas direction across groups was random (Fig. 4.7). Transitions between states were saltatory over changing noise and density. Although the authors appear most interested in the case where coherent motion across the population was produced, their results are interesting from a biological point of view because of the transition from ultimate individuality to well-defined groups. This paper echoes the much simpler work of Inagaki *et al.* (1976) who also explored the relationship between random force and the tendency for groups to form.

What actual fish do

Simulations and models are attractive, in part, because of the intractability of following live fish in schools for biologically realistic time intervals (i.e. longer than seconds). However, despite logistical difficulties, several studies have measured aspects of schooling metrics against which simulation output could be tested. In an incredible paper that currently suffers from the '20-year rule' (that all old papers must become irrelevant and therefore not cited), Partridge (1981) measured relative three-dimensional positions for 20–30 fish schools of adult saithe (*Pollachius virens*) swimming in an annular tank. Among the many relevant findings in this paper were the results that correlation between the heading of fish *i* and its nearest neighbour was low, whereas correlation with neighbour speed was much higher. Lateral neighbours displayed the highest synchrony, followed by neighbours in front. Nearest neighbours exerted the most influence, with significant discounting of farther neighbours, although this damping was not functionally quantified. Finally, above a minimum school size of 15 fish, subgroups, defined by higher than expected correlation in speed and/or heading rather than strict geographic proximity, formed. Occasionally, the differential velocity of the subgroups resulted in local structure breakdown, referred to as lacunae. In fact, these may be the same as the vacuoles that open as a result of local polarity breakdowns in larger schools of clupeids (Fréon *et al.*, 1992). Partridge (1981) suggested that: (1) speed matching is a likely mechanism producing school structure; (2) subgroups may result from a threshold in cognitive capacity as group size grows (that is, the inability for individuals to pay

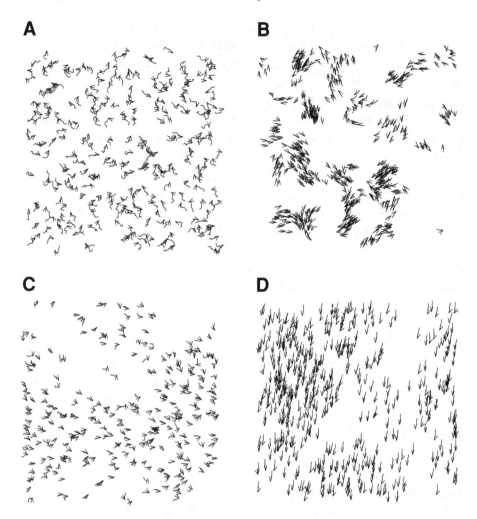

Figure 4.7 Particle velocity (arrow) and trajectory (arrow stem) from a sum-of-forces agent-based simulation varying particle density and noise (error in resultant velocity). (A) starting conditions; (B) low density and noise – small, coherent groups moving in random directions; (C) high density and noise – no coherent groups, some population-level direction correlation; (D) high density and low noise – all particles align, but no groups form. From Viscek *et al.* (1995); reprinted with permission.

attention to all neighbours); and (3) because subgroups are dispersed throughout the school, sudden transitions in velocity could be quickly transmitted throughout the entire school (rather than from nearest neighbour to nearest neighbour). This last point suggests that schools, or subgroups within schools, may act as 'small-world' networks (*sensu* Watts and Strogatz 1998).

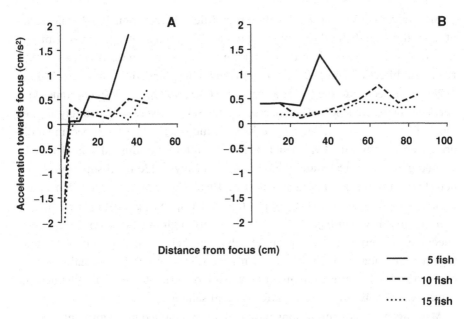

Figure 4.8 Relationship between the acceleration component in the direction of (A) nearest neighbour and (B) school centroid as a function of distance to those entities, and size of the group. Positive values are towards and negative values are away. Redrawn from Parrish and Turchin (1997).

Using multiple video cameras, Parrish and Turchin (1997) were able to follow individual fish in small schools (5–15 fish) of blacksmith (*Chromis punctipinnis*) for 10-second intervals, and used the *x, y, z, t* data to explore the component of acceleration of fish *i* in the direction of suspected foci of attraction. Although noise in the system was extremely high (that is, the fish were not lock-step schoolers), there were two significant attractors: the nearest neighbour, as was also demonstrated by Partridge (1981); and the group as a whole (measured as the centroid). These results were used to produce attraction–repulsion curves as a function of distance from the modelled source (Fig. 4.8). While fish were strongly repulsed from nearest neighbours at less than a body length, attraction to both neighbours and the group as a whole increased steadily at greater distances. Furthermore, the intensity of the attraction was muted in larger (with 15 as opposed to 5 fish) groups. Parrish and Turchin (1997) suggested that individuals in or adjacent to small groups may physically be able to sense and compute the movements of all individuals, whereas individuals in larger groups may use density as a proxy (see also Morton *et al.*, 1994). Using the density rule, stragglers, or those individuals divorced from a group, would head for the middle of a two-dimensional projection, the point approximated by the centroid.

More recently, Viscido *et al.* (2005) quantified three-dimensional trajectories of four- and eight-fish schools of giant danios (*Danio aequipinnatus*) over 5-minute intervals, using stereo digital videography and a computerised tracking algorithm. Architectures ranged from completely non-polarised (i.e. a 'swarm': Shaw, 1978) to perfectly aligned (i.e. a 'school': Shaw, 1978), with steep transitions between these states (*sensu* Couzin *et al.*, 2002). Schools were very strongly aligned most of the time, with irregular periods during which the school became a disorganized swarm (Fig. 4.9A). For real fish, therefore, an aligned school may be a self-organised critical state, which is dynamically stable until something happens to destroy the organisation (Bak *et al.*, 1988; Wu and David, 2002). Simulated groups of eight fish showed the opposite pattern, spending most of their time as a disorganised swarm (Fig. 4.9B). Therefore, although our behavioral rules were adequate to capture some aspects of schooling behaviour (e.g. schools staying together for long periods of time, with stray individuals occasionally becoming 'lost'), clearly some component is missing or needs to be refined before our simulated schools will behave more like real schools.

Many agent-based simulations have explicitly included an alignment force in order to realise the polarity so apparent in fish schools, and measurable here (e.g. Viscido *et al.*, 2005). Both simulations (e.g. Reuter and Breckling, 1994; Couzin *et al.*, 2002) and dynamic models (e.g. Niwa, 1994) have implicitly or explicitly alluded to the sensitivity of alignment inclusion. Essentially, a little goes a long way. Viscido *et al.* (2005) found that time-averaged polarity of real fish schools was most similar to simulated schools when alignment force was 1–5% of the attraction–repulsion force (Fig. 4.10). For simulated schools, very strong alignment forces led to schools that were 'hyper-polarised' (perfectly aligned for long periods), whereas weaker alignment forces led to disorganised swarming as the primary social behaviour. Clearly, some balance of forces exists that will lead to a more natural-looking architecture which still allows for both position shifting within the group, and fission–fusion among groups; however, this balance remains to be discovered.

Although the number of studies and size of the schools over which data are collected have both been small, several generalisations can be made. First, small groups appear to differ quantitatively from larger ones. For instance, dyads are mostly leader–follower (Partridge 1980) and tend to remain planar, whereas fish schools of four or more are increasingly heterogeneous in both elevation and bearing (Partridge 1980). However, even as the group becomes more three-dimensional, the envelope around each fish is not symmetrical, but resembles instead a flattened sphere; that is, fish are closer in z than in xy (Pitcher and Partridge, 1979). Beyond some fairly small threshold, subgroups may appear (Partridge, 1981). Within the school, fish pay most attention to their nearest

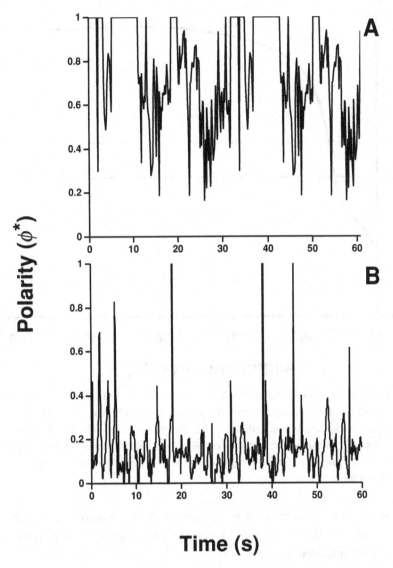

Figure 4.9 Polarity of (A) a real and (B) a simulated school of eight fish over 60 seconds. Here, $\phi^* = 1.0$ represents perfect alignment, and $\phi^* = 0.0$ represents maximum disarray.

neighbour (Partridge *et al.*, 1980; Partridge, 1981; Parrish and Turchin, 1997) followed by some sense of the entire group (Parrish and Turchin, 1997). Fish tend to match speed over position or heading (Partridge, 1981; Doustari and Sannomiya, 1995). A definite school structure (measured as degree of polarisation) appears to be the base state, but is easily destroyed by the individual actions of school members (Viscido *et al.*, 2005). Finally, it is important to remember that

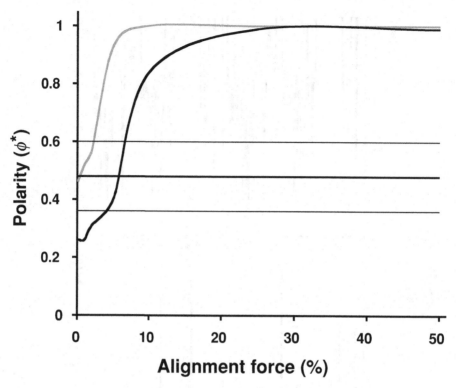

Figure 4.10 Mean group polarity (ϕ^*) as a function of the percentage alignment force in simulation, as compared with the polarity of real fish. Here, $\phi^* = 1.0$ represents perfect alignment, and $\phi^* = 0.0$ represents maximum disarray. Results are shown for simulations of four (grey curve) and eight (black curve) fish. The mean (bold straight line) ± 1 SD (thin straight lines) for real four- and eight-fish schools are shown for comparison.

only as technology allows us to track more individuals over longer intervals of time will we truly be able to generalise emergent phenomena and adequately compare real and simulated datasets.

What is probably important, rule-wise

Obviously, imposing unknowable calculations on individuals is unrealistic. Thus, individuals who know the velocity of the group (e.g. Balchen, 1972), are attracted to a centroid (e.g. Forcardi, 1987; Reynolds, 1987), head directly towards their nearest neighbour when outside the attraction zone (Huth and Wissel, 1992) or all aim towards a point in space (e.g. Reynolds, 1987) will display aggregation, even if these values can not be calculated in life. Morton *et al.* (1994) suggested that individuals may not even be able to calculate reliably the distance to a relatively small set of neighbours ($n = 5$–9); however, fish may be able to sense relative differences in density. Such a rule is almost as efficient at producing aggregations as the more computationally intensive distance to n nearest neighbours. The great strength of an agent-based approach is in the very exploration of only local rules summing to group pattern (Parrish and Edelstein-Keshet, 1999). Similarly, unrealistic constraints, such as preset speed (e.g. Viscek et al., 1995; Stöcker, 1999; Couzin, et al., 2002) will do little to explain actual phenomena, even if the simulations appear to mimic reality.

The type of social forces included, their functional shape and their relative weighting greatly influence all aspects of individual, group and population-level pattern (Parrish et al., 2002). Shape of the attraction–repulsion function can have a significant impact on aggregation dynamics (Warburton and Lazarus, 1991; Parrish et al., 2002), and the few studies of real fish indicate that asymptotic functions with steep repulsion functions may be the norm (Parrish and Turchin, 1997), at least for small schools. Many agent-based simulations have shown aggregation, but only those including alignment, either as an explicit force (e.g. Aoki, 1982; Reuter and Breckling, 1994; Couzin et al., 2002) or implicitly via leaders that others follow (e.g. Gueron et al., 1996), have shown polarity.

Breder (1954) suggested that rather than always count the number of influential neighbours, a two-dimensional projected area might be used, presaging the density assessment rule of Morton et al. (1994). This prediction explains why fish asked to choose between two large groups (e.g. 64 versus 128 fish) spent equal amounts of time with both schools (Nakamura, 1952, as cited in Breder, 1954), whereas fish asked to choose between small groups of different size (e.g. two versus four) could easily do so (Nakamura, 1952; Hager and Helfman, 1991; Krause and Godin, 1994). Finally, recent work suggests that in weakly schooling but gregarious fish, individuals can learn and remember the performance of up to 50 individuals (Griffiths and Magurran, 1997), and make associational decisions accordingly, suggesting that some aspect of neighbour influence may be predetermined (e.g. associate with known poor competitors: Metcalfe and Thompson, 1995). Thus, it is clear that some aspect of local rules may be individual-specific (e.g. fish i choosing to associate with fish j), whereas others may remain extremely general (e.g. fish i choosing to swim towards a higher-density sector).

The number of neighbours considered, and the relative weighting of their influence, is of obvious importance in regulating most aspects of schooling group properties. And while it is probably not possible to discern the exact rule(s) used in nature (Levin, 1999), it may be possible to rule out (or in) possibilities. For instance, it is unlikely that individuals are omniscient (e.g. Reuter and Breckling, 1994; Romey, 1996). Simply on practical grounds, the visual signals that real fish are likely to use in assessing response (e.g. angular velocity of a fixed point on the neighbour, rate of change of solid angle subtended by the neighbour, or optical specification of the time to collision: Dill *et al.*, 1997) can only be calculated accurately for those fish clearly in view (that is, not occluded by others). Thus, a 25–100-body-length zone of attraction is manifestly unrealistic. Reynolds (1987) pointed out that real fish must have a 'constant time algorithm' for deciding direction and velocity. In other words, individuals need a way to minimise, or at least cap, the number of influential neighbours such that larger groups do not lead to ever more computational time resulting in increased decision latency; hesitation can be fatal. This means that either there is a discrete rule (pay attention to *x* neighbours), a dynamic rule (pay attention to *x* neighbours given *y* condition), or a non-neighbour-number rule (assess *z* volume). Although extending neighbour influence throughout the group has appeared to allow a studied consideration of within-group patterns, it has had the improbable effect of never allowing individuals to leave. In other words, the group equals the population, clearly an unrealistic assumption.

Things that need exploring

The majority of agent-based models of fish schooling have examined rule space over which group-level pattern – edges, polarity, structures – emerge (e.g. Reuter and Breckling, 1994; Couzin *et al.*, 2002; Couzin and Krause, 2003) and are stable (Hiramatsu *et al.*, 2000). Stability is an attractive concept, but not useful in its extreme – phalanx structures in which assembled individuals do not rearrange. The problem with this approach is that in the real world, and even in the laboratory, fish join and leave groups constantly. Rule sets need to be explored that allow individuals to shift location within the school, rather than simply aggregate and remain in a static configuration. What rules would allow individuals to: (1) switch positions within the volume of the school, (2) leave the school only to immediately rejoin it and (3) leave the school and search for another group? These common behaviours of schooling fish suggest that there may even be multiple rule sets that an individual can switch on and off as needed. In the next generation of agent-based schooling simulations, rule sets must allow a simultaneous exploration of individual movements provoking group-level pattern and fission–fusion of groups (from stragglers to larger groups). Related to this point, we need trajectories of real fish in schools over long enough time intervals to explore the degree to which all individuals cycle through group positions, or not. Until we know what real fish are doing, it will remain difficult to impossible to ground-truth our simulations.

Group behaviour is a dynamic battle between conformity and selfishness (Parrish and Edelstein-Keshet, 1999). All individuals seek to take selfish advantage, but total individuality would (probably) destroy group structure. To date, most agent-based simulations have concentrated on the emergence of pattern, and not on the expression of individuality. Thus, other than token stochasticity introduced via gamma distributions of variation in speed and/or direction (see Parrish *et al.* (2002) for a review), agents are identical. However, both simulations and experiments have indicated that groups composed of individuals with differing internal states can have significant effects on group size, structure and stability (Romey, 1995, 1996). Simulations on the edge of criticality are needed. In fact, this is a region of rule space where agent-based models can shed light on conformity constraints imposed by group membership.

Can local rules dictate group size, independent of the maximum size dictated by resource limitation? Several agent-based simulations have suggested that rule sets, especially the number of influential neighbours, and starting conditions, especially the population size, can have a profound influence on resulting group size (Couzin *et al.*, 2002; Parrish *et al.*, 2002; Viscido *et al.*, unpubl. data). Group size scaling as a function of population size has been demonstrated in a range of organisms, including fish (Bonabeau *et al.*, 1999). On the other hand, optimality models clearly predict that individuals should join or leave groups as a function of individual benefit, creating a set of groups at or near critical group size (Sibly, 1983). When asked to choose, real fish will most often select larger groups (Krause and Godin, 1994), although they cannot always discern differences between similarly sized larger groups (Hager and Helfman, 1991). Agent-based simulations at truly large population sizes and with a realistic number of influential neighbours are needed to explore the relationship between population size, group size and the number of influential neighbours.

To date, our limited three-dimensional datasets on actual schools have been produced (necessarily) in the laboratory under very artificial conditions, and with small schools. Do these patterns and the simulations we use to explore potential local rule sets to explain them – hold in the real world where schools of clupeids (herring, sardine, pilchard) exceed millions of fish per school? Acoustic analysis indicates that large free-swimming schools have complex amoeboid shapes, often containing areas of no fish (vacuoles: Fréon *et al.*, 1992) and superdense regions (nuclei: F. Gerlotto, pers. comm.), both of which appear ephemeral. Packing density in herring schools can vary by two orders of magnitude (Misund and Floen, 1993). Finally, schools are themselves fluid entities, where membership may change quickly (Hilborn, 1991) even if school size and other functional attributes remain constant. Thus, the degree of regularity in architecture and membership exhibited by many simulations may represent our concept of a school, rather than the actuality. At the very least, simulations must be robust to disturbance (e.g. obstacles, predators, change in sensory fields, erratic behaviour of individual agents) such that we can discern under what range of conditions schools will persist, rather than dissolve. This latter examination is different, we believe, from the exploration of rule space over which aggregation predominates given no other forcing (e.g. Fig. 4.5; Couzin *et al.*, 2002).

Conclusions

Agent-based approaches to the study of fish schooling have allowed us to explore local rule sets, and the associated parameter space, within which aggregation and schooling might occur. Unlike any set of laboratory or field experiments, the computational approach has the potential to examine systematically the multiple adaptive peaks in the landscape of three-dimensional aggregation, pointing the way towards which rules are necessary, even fundamental. The downside is that many models explore only a small portion of the state space, include unrealistic rules, or fail to ground-truth results against actual data. Finally, agent-based approaches need to expand to incorporate the internal state of the agents. Knowing the traffic rules is important, but there must be an underlying set of proximate and ultimate reasons for the aggregation to exist, and persist. These shortcomings need to be addressed if agent-based modelling, and the more general study of self-organisation, are to become part of the mainstream of biology.

Acknowledgements

The authors would like to thank C. Hemelrijk, J. Krause and an anonymous reviewer for reading and improving the manuscript. D. Grünbaum wrote the tracking code allowing us to obtain the three-dimensional fish trajectory data highlighted in Fig. 4.9 and 4.10. I. McFarland and J. Weitzman tracked fish. The authors were supported in part by a National Science Foundation grant (CCR-9980058) to J. Parrish and D. Grünbaum.

References

Aoki, I. (1982). A simulation study on the schooling mechanism in fish. *Bull. Japan. Soc. Sci. Fish.* **48**, 1081–1088.

(1984). Internal dynamics of fish schools in relation to inter-fish distance. *Bull. Japan. Soc. Sci. Fish.* **50**, 751–758.

Bak, P., Tang, C. and Wiesenfeld, K. (1988). Self-organised criticality. *Phys. Rev. A* **38**, 364–374.

Bakun, A. and Cury, P. (1999). The 'school trap': a mechanism promoting large-amplitude out-of-phase population oscillations of small pelagic fish species. *Ecol. Lett.* **2**, 349–351.

Balchen, J. G. (1972). Feedback control of schooling fish. In *Proce. Int. Federation Automatic Control 5th World Congress*, Paper 14.3.

Bonabeau, E., Dagorn, L. and Fréon, P. (1999). Scaling in animal group-size distributions. *Proc. Natl Acad. Sci. USA* **96**, 4472–4477.

Breder, C. M. (1951). Studies on the structure of the fish school. *Bull. Mus. Am. Nat. Hist.* **98**, 1–28.

(1954). Equations descriptive of fish schools and other animal aggregations. *Ecology* **35**, 361–370.

(1976). Fish schools as operational structures. *Fishery Bull.* **74**, 471–502.

Camazine, S., Deneubourg, J. L. and Franks, N. R. (2001). *Self-Organisation in Biological Systems*. Princeton, NJ: Princeton University Press.

Clark, C. W. and Mangel, M. (1984). Foraging and flocking strategies: information in an uncertain environment. *Am. Naturalist* **123**, 626–641.

Couzin, I. D. and Krause, J. (2003). Self-organisation and collective behaviour of vertebrates. *Adv. Study Behav.* **32**, 1–67.

Couzin, I. D., Krause, J., James, R., Ruxton, G. D. and Franks, N. R. (2002). Collective memory and spatial sorting in animal groups. *J. Theoret. Biol.* **218**, 1–11.

Dill, L. M., Holling, C. S. and Palmer, L. H. (1997). Predicting the three-dimensional structure of animal aggregations from functional considerations: the role of information. In *Animal Groups in Three Dimensions*, ed. J. K. Parrish and W. M. Hamner. Cambridge: Cambridge University Press, pp. 207–224.

Doustari, M. A. and Sannomiya, N. (1992). A simulation study on schooling mechanism in fish behavior. *Trans. Inst. Syst. Contr. Inform. Engin.* **5**, 521–523.

(1993a). Autonomous decentralized mechanism in fish behavior model. In *Proc. 1st Int. Symp. Autonomous Decentralized Systems*, Tokyo, pp. 414–420.

(1993b). How does fish school change form? A hypothesis from simulation study. *Trans. Soc. Instr. Contr. Engin.* **29**, 1388–1390.

(1995). A simulation study on schooling behaviour of fish in a water tank. *Int. J. Systems Sci.* **26**, 2295–2308.

Duffy, D. C. and Wissel, C. (1988). Models of fish school size in relation to environmental productivity. *Ecol. Model.* **40**, 201–211.

Forcardi, S. (1987). Foraging and social behaviour of ungulates: proposals for a mathematical model. In *Cognitive Processes and Spatial Orientation in Animal and Man*, ed. P. Ellen and C. Thinus-Blanc. Dordrecht: Martinus Nijhoff, pp. 295–304.

Fréon, P., Gerlotto, F. and Soria, M. (1992). Changes in school structure according to external stimuli: description and influence on acoustic assessment. *Fish. Res.* **15**, 45–66.

Griffiths, S. W. and Magurran, A. E. (1997). Schooling preferences for familiar fish vary with group size in a wild guppy population. *Proc. Roy. Soc. London B* **264**, 547–551.

Gueron, S., Levin, S. A. and Rubenstein, D. I. (1996). The dynamics of herds: from individuals to aggregations. *J. Theoret. Biol.* **182**, 85–98.

Hager, M. C. and Helfman, G. S. (1991). Safety in numbers: shoal size choice by minnows under predatory threat. *Behav. Ecol. Sociobiol.* **29**, 271–276.

Hamilton, W. D. (1971). Geometry for the selfish herd. *J. Theoret. Biol.* **31**, 295–311.

Hamner, W. M. and Parrish, J. K. (1997). Is the sum of the parts equal to the whole: the conflict between individuality and group membership. In *Animal Groups in Three Dimensions*, ed. J. K. Parrish and W. H. Hamner. Cambridge: Cambridge University Press, pp. 163–173.

Helbing, D. and Huberman, B. A. (1998). Coherent moving states in highway traffic. *Nature* **396**, 738–740.

Hemelrijk, C. K. (2000). Towards the integration of social dominance and spatial structure. *Anim. Behav.* **59**, 1035–1048.

Hilborn, R. (1991). Modeling the stability of fish schools: exchange of individual fish between schools of skipjack tuna (*Katsuwonus pelamis*). *Can. J. Fish. Aquat. Sci.* **48**, 1081–1091.

Hiramatsu, K., Shikasho, S. and Mori, K. (2000). Mathematical modeling of fish schooling of Japanese medaka using basic behavioral patterns. *J. Fac. Agric. Kyushu Univ.* **45**, 237–253.

Huth, A. and Wissel, C. (1990). The movement of fish schools: a simulation model. In *Biological Motion*, ed. W. Alt and G. Hoffman. Berlin: Springer-Valag, pp. 578–590.

(1992). The simulation of the movement of fish schools. *J. Theoret. Biol.* **156**, 365–385.

(1994). The simulation of fish schools in comparison with experimental data. *Ecol. Model.* **75**, 135–145.

Inagaki, T., Sakamoto, W. and Kuroki, T. (1976). Studies on the schooling behavior of fish. II. Mathematical modeling of schooling form depending on the intensity of mutual force between individuals. *Bull. Japan. Soc. Sci. Fish.* **42**: 265–270.

James, R., Bennett, P. G. and Krause, J. (2004). Geometry for mutualistic and selfish herds: the limited domain of danger. *J. Theoret. Biol.* **228**, 107–113.

Krause, J. and Godin, J. G. J. (1994). Shoal choice in the banded killifish (*Fundulus diaphanus*, Teleostei, Cyprinodontidae): effects of predation risk, fish size, species composition, and size of shoals. *Ethology* **98**, 128–136.

Krause, J. and Ruxton, G. D. (2002). *Living in Groups*. New York: Oxford University Press.

Kunz, H. and Hemelrijk, C. K. (2003). Artificial fish schools: collective effects of school size, body size, and body form. *Artif. Life* **9**, 237–253.

Levin, S. A. (1999). *Fragile Dominion: Complexity and the Commons*. Reading, MA: Perseus Books.

McFarland, W. M. and Moss, S. A. (1967). Internal behavior in fish schools. *Science* **156**, 260–262.

Metcalfe, N. B. and Thompson, B. C. (1995). Fish recognize and prefer to shoal with poor competitors. *Proc. Roy. Soc. London B* **259**, 207–210.

Misund, O. A. and Floen, S. (1993). Packing density structure of herring schools. *ICES Mar. Sci. Symp.* **196**, 26–29.

Morton, T. L., Haefner, J. W., Nugala, V., Decino, R. D. and Mendes, L. (1994). The Selfish Herd revisited: do simple movement rules reduce relative predation risk? *J. Theoret. Biol.* **167**, 73–79.

Nakamura, Y. (1952). Some experiments of the shoaling reaction in *Oryzias latipes* (Temminck et Schlegel). *Bull. Japan. Soc. Sci. Fish.* **18**, 93–101.

Niwa, H. S. (1994). Self-organizing dynamics model of fish schooling. *J. Theoret. Biol.* **171**, 123–136.

Nonacs, P., Smith, P. E. and Mangel, M. (1998). Modeling foraging in the northern anchovy (*Engraulis mordax*): individual behavior can predict school dynamics and population biology. *Can. J. Fish. Aquat. Sci.* **55**, 1179–1188.

Nøttestad, L. and Axelsen, B. E. (1999). Herring schooling manoeuvres in response to killer whale attacks. *Can. J. Zool.* **77**, 1540–1546.

Parr, A. (1927). A contribution on the theoretical analysis of the schooling behavior of fishes. *Occ. Papers Bingham Oceanogr. Coll.* **1**, 1–32.

Parrish, J. K. (1989). Re-examining the selfish herd: are central fish safer? *Anim. Behav.* **38**, 1048–1053.

(1992). Levels of diurnal predation on a school of flat-iron herring, *Harengula thrissina*. *Envir. Biol. Fish.* **24**, 257–263.

Parrish, J. K. and Edelstein-Keshet, L. (1999). Complexity, pattern, and evolutionary trade-offs in animal aggregation. *Science* **284**, 99–101.

(2000). Reply to Danchin and Wagner. *Science* **287**, 804–805.

Parrish, J. K. and Turchin, P. (1997). Individual decisions, traffic rules, and emergent pattern in schooling fish. In *Animal Groups in Three Dimensions*, ed. J. K. Parrish and W. M. Hamner. Cambridge: Cambridge University Press, pp. 126–141.

Parrish, J. K., Viscido, S. V. and Grunbaum, D. (2002). Self-organized fish schools: an examination of emergent properties. *Biol. Bull.* **202**, 296–305.

Partridge, B. L. (1980). The effect of school size on the structure and dynamics of minnow schools. *Anim. Behav.* **28**, 68–77.

(1981). Internal dynamics and the interrelations of fish in schools. *J. Comp. Physiol.* **144A**, 313–325.

Partridge, B. L., Pitcher, T., Cullen, J. M. and Wilson, J. K. (1980). The three-dimensional structure of fish schools. *Behav. Ecol. Sociobiol.* **6**, 277–288.

Pitcher, T. J. and Parrish, J. K. (1993). Functions of shoaling behaviour in teleosts. In *Behaviour of Teleost Fishes*, 2nd edn, ed. T. J. Pitcher. London: Chapman and Hall, pp. 363–479.

Pitcher, T. J. and Partridge, B. L. (1979). Fish school density and volume. *Marine Biol.* **54**, 383–394.

Reuter, H. and Breckling, B. (1994). Self-organization of fish schools: an object-oriented model. *Ecol. Model.* **75/76**, 147–159.

Reynolds, C. W. (1987). Flocks, herds, and schools: a distributed behavioral model. *Comput. Graph.* **21**, 25–33.

Romey, W. L. (1995). Position preferences within groups: do whirligigs select positions which balance feeding opportunities with predator avoidance? *Behav. Ecol. Sociobiol.* **37**, 195–200.

(1996). Individual differences make a difference in the trajectories of simulated schools of fish. *Ecol. Model.* **92**, 65–77.

Sakai, S. (1973). A model for group structure and its behavior. *Biophysics* **13**, 82–90. (In Japanese).

Sannomiya, N. and Doustari, M. A. (1996). A simulation study on autonomous decentralized mechanism in fish behaviour model. *Int. J. Systems Sci.* **27**, 1001–1007.

Sannomiya, N. and Matuda, K. (1984). A mathematical model of fish behavior in a water tank. IEEE *Trans. Systems, Man and Cybernetics* **14**, 157–162.

Sannomiya, N., Nakamine, H. and Matuda, K. (1990). Application of system theory to modeling of fish behavior. In *Proc. 29th IEEE Conf. Decision and Control*, vol. 5, pp. 2793–2799.

Shaw, E. (1978). Schooling fishes. *Am. Sci.* **66**, 166–175.

Sibly, R. M. (1983). Optimal group size is unstable. *Anim. Behav.* **31**, 947–948.

Steinbeck, J. and Ricketts, E. (1941). *The Log from the Sea of Cortez*. New York: Viking Press.

Stöcker, S. (1999). Models for tuna school formation. *Math. Biosci.* **156**, 167–190.

Vabø, R. and Nøttestad, L. (1997). An individual-based model of fish school reactions: predicting antipredator behaviour as observed in nature. *Fish. Oceanogr.* **6**, 155–171.

Van Olst, J. C. and Hunter, J. R. (1970). Some aspects of the organization of fish schools. *J. Fish. Res. Board Canada* **27**, 1225–1238.

Viscek, T., Czirok, A., Ben-Jacob, E. and Eshocet, O. (1995). Novel type of phase transition in a system of self-driven particles. *Phys. Rev. Lett.* **75**, 1226–1229.

Viscido, S. V., Parrish, J. K. and Grünbaum, D. (2005). Individual behavior and emergent properties of fish schools: a comparison of observation and theory. *Ecol. Model.*

Warburton, K. and Lazarus, J. (1991). Tendency–distance models of social cohesion in animal groups. *J. Theoret. Biol.* **150**, 473–488.

Watts, D. J. and Strogatz, S. H. (1998). Collective dynamics of 'small-world' networks. *Nature* **393**, 440–442.

Weihs, D. (1973). Hydromechanics of fish schooling. *Nature* **241**, 290–294.

 (1975). Some hydrodynamical aspects of fish schooling. In *Swimming and Flying in Nature*, ed. T. Y. Wu, C. J. Broklaw and C. Brennan. New York: Plenum Press, pp. 703–718.

Williams, G. C. (1966). *Adaptation and Natural Selection*. Princeton, NJ: Princeton University Press.

Wilson, E. O. (1975). *Sociobiology: The New Synthesis*. Cambridge, MA: Harvard University Press.

Wu, J. and David, J. L. (2002). A spatially explicit hierarchical approach to modeling complex ecological systems: theory and applications. *Ecol. Model.* **153**, 7–26.

5

A process-oriented approach to the social behaviour of primates

CHARLOTTE K. HEMELRIJK

University of Groningen

Introduction

The marked complexity of primate social behaviour is usually ascribed to the extraordinary intelligence of primates (Whiten and Byrne, 1986, 1997; Byrne and Whiten, 1988). Of the 'social tools' adopted by primates various forms of 'bargaining' or exchange relationship (such as the interchange of grooming for received support as supposed for chimpanzees) have drawn much attention in both cognitive and evolutionary studies. Exchange relationships are often assumed to account for the occurrence of sociopositive acts, because these acts, such as grooming, food-sharing and support in fights by primates, seem to lower the fitness of the actor and to enhance that of the receiver. The theories that are commonly applied to explain such acts are based on the assumption that the tendency to display non-selfish behaviour (so-called 'altruism') is genetically encoded. For each aspect, on the basis of cost–benefit arguments, separate adaptive explanations are given and separate acts are supposed to contribute independently to the fitness of an individual (so that the complete fitness of an individual equals the sum of the contributions of the separate traits). The three main theories are:

(1) The kin selection theory (Hamilton, 1964). Altruism may be spreading evolutionarily if it is directed towards kin, because of the high probability that closely related individuals share the gene responsible for its realisation.

Self-Organisation and Evolution of Social Systems, ed. Charlotte K. Hemelrijk.
Published by Cambridge University Press. © Cambridge University Press 2005.

(2)   The theory of reciprocal altruism (Trivers, 1971). Altruism can be part of a cooperative relationship, if it is returned by the receiver to the actor. Although the altruist suffers a loss in the short term, by being 'paid back' later, he will benefit in the long run.

(3)   The sexual selection theory (Darwin, 1871; Trivers, 1971) explains altruistic behaviour to females as a male reproductive strategy to win matings. The theory presupposes that females should prefer mating with their male beneficiaries to males from whom they receive no (or fewer) such services.

Whereas these theories may explain certain facts of primate life, they do not explain all facts and that is why an additional framework for studying behaviour is needed. We will show how a more dynamic kind of explanation that comprises the effect of the behavioural circumstances is also possible. It will be shown that the same behavioural rules under different circumstances lead to different behavioural phenomena. Further, patterns may arise that are not coded in the behavioural rules, but emerge from the interactions among the agents by self-organisation. In this way a new kind of explanation is generated. To derive such hypotheses and explanations, certain kinds of computer models are of great help.

More specifically, we will show how our own empirical findings of sociopositive behaviour among chimpanzees cannot be explained by the traditional theories mentioned above as exchange of sociopositive behaviour for copulations or for offspring (pp. 83–84). Therefore, we turn to a more context-oriented approach (pp. 84–87). We include in our theories the effects of competition (whether for food, mates and safe spatial positions does not matter) on sociopositive relationships. For instance, for grooming behaviour, we will show with data from real primates how the degree of reciprocation varies markedly with the circumstances, namely the sex ratio of a group and the presence of one or more males in a group. Thus, we ascribe differences in degree of grooming reciprocation to the same behavioural response under different social conditions. This contrasts with traditional theories in which these would be ascribed rather to specifically selected behavioural rules inbuilt to modify behaviour when the group composition changes, or where they would be attributed to inherent differences between typical single and multi-male species. In the last section of this chapter (pp. 87–100), we will show how the dynamics of competitive interactions in an artificial society gives rise to certain kinds of self-organised patterns. It will appear that these self-organised patterns may influence sociopositive behaviour as a side effect, in such a way that under some conditions patterns arise that do indeed look like exchange, but which arise in a completely different way. These phenomena will then lead to new hypotheses about reciprocation and exchange and about many other aspects of the social behaviour of real primates (and other animals).

The traditional theories: exchange of sociopositive behaviour

At first sight many aspects of the social behaviour of chimpanzees seem to fit traditional theories of kin selection, sexual selection and reciprocal altruism, but on closer observation the evidence appears weak. Let's take three examples.

First, male chimpanzees have been observed cooperatively to attack solitary males of neighbouring communities (Goodall, 1986). Because in a 'female-transfer' species, the females move to neighbouring communities when they grow up, it has been argued that in the course of time males become more and more related to each other. This is why cooperative relationships among male chimpanzees are generally attributed to kinship (e.g. see Goodall, 1986). However, several DNA-typing studies of a natural chimpanzee colony in Kibale (Goldberg and Wrangham, 1997; Merriwether et al., 2000; Mitani et al., 2002) revealed that cooperating males were not more closely related to each other than indifferent (non-cooperative) ones.

Second, chimpanzee males have been seen to reciprocate support in conflicts among themselves (de Waal, 1978). This was initially regarded as a case of reciprocal altruism in which, after receiving benefits, individual chimpanzees feel a 'moral' obligation to pay back (de Waal and Luttrell, 1989). They are supposed to keep track of the number of acts received from every partner. However, in our extensive study of reciprocation, we have found that males appear to reciprocate only in periods without a clear-cut alpha-male (Hemelrijk and Ek, 1991), and not when the position of the alpha-male is strong. As an alternative, simpler explanation we suggest that males may join in one another's fights to attack common rivals and that this leads to seeming reciprocity in the data. In such opportunistic strategies, the supporting behaviour is wholly selfish and there is no need to keep records. Direct selfishness is also in line with the results of our study of communicative gestures that seem to function as requests to others (known as 'side-directed behaviour': de Waal and van Hooff, 1981); no connection between reciprocation and complying with requests from others could be demonstrated (Hemelrijk et al., 1991).

Third, males seem to render services to females, such as grooming, supporting them in conflicts and sharing food with them (Teleki, 1973; Tutin, 1980; Goodall, 1986; Stanford, 1996). Yet we have not found any evidence that male services to females served as a reproductive strategy as is expected if we apply the theory of sexual selection (Trivers, 1971). Although several studies suggest that sociopositive relations between males and females are associated with fitness benefits, in our detailed statistical analysis copulation frequency was not found to be correlated with affiliative acts, such as support and food sharing, and only few correlations with grooming behaviour were observed (Hemelrijk et al., 1992). However, grooming may simply facilitate mating by suppressing aggression in males and a tendency to flee in females, and thus it may be part of the sexual repertoire rather than being an exchange for mating opportunities. Furthermore, the frequency of copulation of a male does not correlate significantly with the number of his offspring (Meier et al., 2000) and therefore cannot be used as an indication of fitness. All this makes it unlikely that exchange actually occurs at the behavioural level. However, this does not rule out possible fitness benefits. It remains possible that inter-sexual sociopositive behaviour may affect the production of offspring via some physical, post-copulatory choice mechanism in females (Martin, 1992). In line with the previous results, we found, however, no support for this notion of trade either in our study of affiliation in exchange for fitness benefits (using paternity inferences from microsatellite analyses: Meier et al., 2000) or in our investigations of copulation frequency (Hemelrijk et al., 1999). First, males did not sire more offspring with females they groomed more frequently, or supported more often or with whom they shared food more frequently. Correspondingly, females did not give birth to more offspring sired by males from whom they received more services. Further, males that were more cooperative with females in general (regardless of female identity) did not sire more progeny. A possible shortcoming of this study is that the colony may not be representative of a chimpanzee community because of its captive condition. However, our results agree with findings under natural conditions, where chimpanzees are described as highly promiscuous (e.g. Goodall, 1986; Morin, 1993; Wallis, 1997; Constable et al., 2001).

Because of the general absence of fitness benefits accruing to sociopositive behaviour not only in chimpanzees, but also in several other species of primates (e.g. Menard et al., 1992; Paul et al., 1992; Jurke et al., 1995), we must turn to a more system-oriented perspective in which we study sociopositive behaviour as an *integral* part of the species' social structure.

The introduction of context: sex ratio and philopatry

An important feature of the social structure of primate societies is the identity of the migrating sex, i.e. which of the sexes migrates and which is philopatric (Pusey and Packer, 1987). In some species females migrate to other groups when adult (so-called female-transfer or male-resident species), but more often males are the migrating sex and females remain in their native group for life (female-resident species).

Wrangham (1980) describes relationships among individuals of the philopatric sex as 'bonded' and those in the migrating sex as indifferent, and this difference in bonding is explained by the difference in the degree of kinship among the individuals of the resident and migrating sex. To verify the suggested difference in bonding between the resident and migrating sex, we have collected from publications social interaction matrices of grooming of 14 primate species (Hemelrijk and Luteijn, 1998). As a measurement method of the degree of social bonding, we use the degree of reciprocation of grooming at a group level as has been described by Hemelrijk (1990a, b). In line with Wrangham's description, the degree of grooming reciprocation is stronger in the resident than the migrating sex. Thus, we conclude that this may be used as an estimate of bonding.

Another argument of evolutionary theory is that females may also benefit from building up (social and sexual) relationships with resident males, because such relationships protect females against other males. This may be particularly important for female-resident species, because, when males immigrate into a new group, they sometimes kill newborn infants (van Schaik, 1989). Because some males may be better protectors than others, we assumed that females would compete for social relationships with certain males and that this could harm 'social bonding' among females. If so, female social relationships should deteriorate more, the lower the male/female ratio (i.e. the socionomic sex ratio) of the group is. This reasoning does not hold for female-transfer species, for two reasons. First, in female-transfer species females may migrate to groups with a more favourable sex ratio, and second, relationships among females are supposed to be indifferent (Wrangham, 1980).

In accordance with this, our analysis actually shows that reciprocation is independent of sex ratio in female-transfer species, and in female-resident species females manifest a stronger reciprocation of grooming at higher socionomic sex ratios. Unexpectedly, the effect of sex ratio on the degree of reciprocation was stronger in typical single-male (according to the number of females present) than in multi-male species; for single-male species the regression line is much steeper than for multi-male species (see regression lines of Fig. 5.1).

The question is whether this difference in slope reflects an inherent difference between single- and multi-male species or if it is a direct effect of the presence of one or more males in a group. To establish this we looked for data (in publications) of single-male groups of species that typically live in multi-male groups under natural conditions (such as rhesus and Japanese macaques). After plotting these together with the regression lines already inferred from previous data (Fig. 5.1), it appeared that points of single-male groups fell around the line

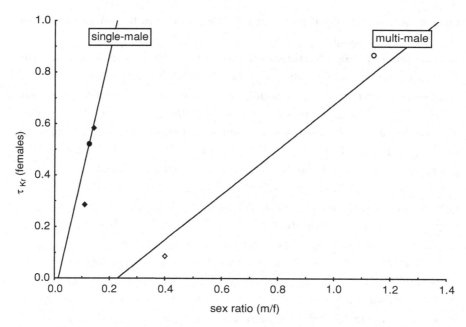

Figure 5.1 Socionomic sex ratio and degree of grooming reciprocation among females. Regression lines are calculated from data (not shown) on single-male and multi-male species under natural conditions. Additional data points are from captive single- and multi-male groups from the same species. Open circle: *Macaca fuscata* (Furuichi, 1985); open diamond: *M. fascicularis* (Huysmans, unpubl. data); solid circle: *M. fuscata* (Mehlman and Chapais, 1988); solid diamonds: *M. fascicularis* (Butovskaya *et al.*, 1995).

for single-male species, and for multi-male groups along the line of multi-male species.

This means that the difference in slope between the lines should be interpreted as a direct effect of the presence of one versus more males in a group. This remarkable outcome casts light upon the question how such competition comes about. In multi-male groups dominant males interfere in the social interactions between subordinate males and females and consequently, in such groups males are less often available per time unit for interactions with females. Therefore, for the same sex ratio, females in multi-male groups have to compete more strongly for males (and consequently, reciprocate grooming less) than in single-male groups. Furthermore, in multi-male groups competition among females diminishes only slightly when the number of males per female increases, because this increase of the relative number of males intensifies competition among males for females and this leads to increased intervention of inter-sexual relationships by rival males. In other words, the decrease in competition among females due to a reduced sex ratio is partly counterbalanced by increased competition among males for females. This explains why females increase their reciprocation with rising sex ratio at a slower rate in multi-male groups than in single-male groups.

The crucial difference between the more traditional comparative studies and ours is that in our study the contrast in behaviour among females between single- and multi-male groups is supposed to reflect nothing more than *different opportunities* for interactions. To explain this variability of behaviour we do not assume an additional component of intelligence, as for instance Hamilton and Bulger (1992) do. These authors regard variation in male behaviour between single- and multi-male groups as a specific adaptive behavioural response to different group compositions and as a sign of 'intelligence'. Our results might also be interpreted likewise, i.e. that females adapt their behaviour specifically to the presence of one or more males in a group, but such a cognitive assumption is superfluous. What we have found is, we believe, purely a consequence of females applying one and the same set of rules, which leads to different results due to the variation in their opportunities to interact with males.

Let us now turn to a certain type of modelling that is very useful for generating such hypotheses about effects of varying behavioural opportunities and that shows that patterns may arise by self-organisation.

Modelling: complex social behaviour from simple rules

Whereas demography may change behavioural opportunities and thus affect social behaviour, social behaviour may also change the (social) environment and the changed environment may in turn influence social behaviour. Such positive feedback may lead to behavioural patterns by self-organisation in the absence of specific behavioural rules for these patterns.

A self-organising approach to explain patterns observed at the level of a group has already been advocated implicitly by Hinde (1982). He distinguishes four different levels of complexity within a society (i.e. individual behaviour, interactions, relationships and social structure), each having its own emergent properties. Each level is described in terms of the lower level, and levels are supposed to influence each other mutually. This means that, for example, the nature of the behaviour of the participants influences their relationships, and these relationships in turn affect the participants' behaviour.

From an empirical point of view, however, it is very difficult to distinguish how far higher-level properties emerge as consequences of interactions or are specific individual qualities, and it is here that models can be of great help. The type of models we will discuss here for studying various etho-ecological processes are called individual-oriented, individual-based or 'artificial life' models (e.g. see Judson, 1994) and are also known as MIRROR-worlds (used in studies of bumble-bees: Hogeweg and Hesper, 1983, 1985; and chimpanzee subgroup formation: te Boekhorst and Hogeweg, 1994).

Here we will see how these models are eminently suited to study social relationships among individuals within groups in a simple, individual-oriented model called DomWorld. A model of primate social behaviour must as a minimal condition consist in groups and contain the essentials of competition. A consequence of competition within groups is the development of a dominance hierarchy. Dominance is a hotly debated topic, particularly as regards the way it is acquired. Some suppose that the quality to become high-ranking is inherited (Ellis, 1994), but this is contradicted by the difference in rank positions occupied by the same individual in form–reform experiments (e.g. Bernstein and Gordon, 1980; Dugatkin *et al.*, 1994). It is also at variance with the overwhelming evidence from many animal species, (such as spiders, insects, fishes, amphibians, reptiles and mammals, including humans: see Mazur, 1985; Bonabeau *et al.*, 1996) that winning and losing competitive interactions, besides being partly ruled by chance, has self-reinforcing effects.

This 'winner/loser' effect is the core of an artificial-life model published by Hogeweg (1988). Her model consisted of a homogeneous world inhabited by simple agents equipped with only two qualities: a tendency to aggregate and, upon meeting each other, to perform competitive interactions in which the effects of winning and losing are self-reinforcing. To simulate dominance interactions, Hogeweg gave each agent a dominance value that indicated its chance of winning. When agents met each other they performed a dominance interaction. The outcome of such an interaction depended on the relative dominance values of both partners and chance. After a fight had been decided the loser fled from its opponent and the dominance values of both partners were updated. Losing decreased the dominance value of an agent, victory increased it. These dynamics conformed to a damped positive feedback, because when a lower-ranking opponent was beaten the dominance values of both partners were changed by a smaller amount than when, unexpectedly, a fight with an opponent of lower rank was lost. In the latter case, the change in dominance values of both partners was greater. Thus, although at the beginning of a run all agents started with the same dominance value, a dominance hierarchy emerged and there were indications of a spatial structure with dominants in the centre and subordinates at the periphery. Because dominance hierarchy and spatial structure are found in many animal species, I decided to extend this model in such a way that it could take on specific problems of ethology. As will be shown below, I have shown, for instance, how patterns of reciprocation of help in fights can be produced as an emergent property (pp. 89–90) and how (for certain strategies of attack and intensities of aggression only) with increasing familiarity among

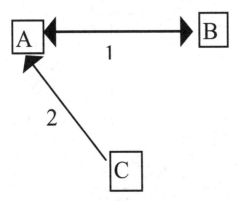

Figure 5.2 Schematic representation of a triadical interaction: (1) fight between A and B; next (2) C attacks A. The behaviour by C is interpreted as 'support' for B.

agents their aggression reduces automatically (pp. 91–93) and a spatial structure with dominants in the centre originates (pp. 93–94).

The emergence of reciprocation of support in conflicts

In the artificial world (called DomWorld) reciprocation of support actually arises and does so in agents that are unable to keep records of acts, do not return debts and lack all motivation to help (Hemelrijk, 1996a): all the same behaviour that looks like helping occurs whenever, by pure chance, agent C attacks another (A), who happens already to be involved in a fight with agent B. Using the same criteria as primatologists do, C is then said to support B against A (Fig. 5.2). In line with my own previous research on chimpanzees, support is considered to be reciprocated whenever agents support more often those partners from whom they receive more support in return (Hemelrijk, 1990a, b).

Supporting behaviour was reciprocated in 50% of the runs of the model and, interestingly, occurs more often in loose than in cohesive groups. This pattern appears to arise from the spatial configuration of agents (Hemelrijk, 1997). Two agents often drive a third into each other's range of attack. In this way they take turns in chasing away the same victim (Fig. 5.3) and thus they seem to 'reciprocate' each other's 'support'. Because cooperating agents are less disturbed and distracted by others in loose groups than in denser ones, reciprocation occurs more frequently and bouts of alternating 'support' last longer in such settings. Looseness of grouping is itself a consequence of the larger radius of attack of the agents. Thus, the unexpected conclusion from the virtual world – and a testable hypothesis for the real world – is that more aggressive agents are more 'cooperative'!

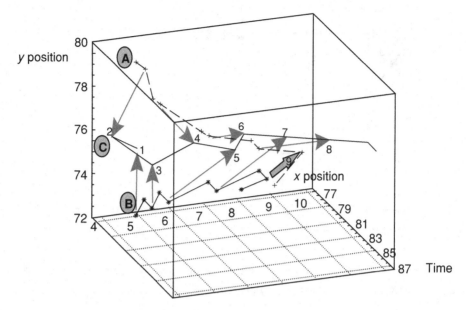

Figure 5.3 Series of events of reciprocation of support among two agents in which A and B alternately attack C. Arrows represent acts of attack, the accompanying numbers indicate time-steps. Note that at the ninth time-step (thick arrow), one of the supporters becomes the victim himself. Units on the time axes are arbitrary numbers of activations in the simulation.

Cooperation by turn-taking as found in my model closely resembles support behaviour observed in male chimpanzees (Hemelrijk and Ek, 1991) and communal hunting by lions. It is also, from an observer's point of view, similar to the famous 'tit-for-tat strategy' in game theory (Axelrod and Hamilton, 1981). However, this agreement questions rather than supports the validity of the assumptions behind the strategy. In a game-theoretical framework cooperation is assumed to evolve on the basis of pay-off benefits in terms of fitness. It is studied as an isolated feature, unconnected to any other behavioural activity, despite the common knowledge that natural selection operates on complete individuals. The present study, in contrast, neither deals with evolutionary processes, nor with pay-offs from cooperation. Instead, cooperation is viewed as a direct consequence of the intertwined effects of local dominance interactions among aggregating agents. This result does not preclude that selection may actually operate on such emergent patterns of cooperation, but this is a question for further study.

This explanation resembles the one proposed by Stephens *et al.* (1997) for the coordinated exploration of predators by sticklebacks. Whereas Milinski (1987) argued that turn-taking by two individuals that are approaching the predator is evidence for a tit-for-tat strategy, Stephens *et al.* (1997) believe that turn-taking is an automatic consequence of the combination of the behavioural tendencies: approaching and shoaling.

Self-organised reduction of aggression

An unrealistic feature of DomWorld is that upon meeting each other, agents invariably attack the opponent. Actually, when real individuals are brought together for the first time, aggression flares only for a limited period and then it declines. This has been empirically established in several animal species (e.g. chickens: Guhl, 1968; primates: Kummer, 1974). The interpretation is that individuals fight to reduce the ambiguity of relationships (Pagel and Dawkins, 1997) and once relationships are clear, fighting should decline to save energy (here called an 'ambiguity-reducing' strategy). On the other hand, it has also been put forward that individuals should continuously strive after a higher rank and should attack always unless it is too dangerous because an opponent is clearly superior (e.g. see Datta and Beauchamp, 1991). In fact, that greater risk of getting seriously wounded reduces aggression is also found by Thierry (1985a): in macaque species in which aggression is intense (often in the form of biting), individuals less often engage in counter-attack than in species with mild aggression (in the form of smacking or hitting).

With the help of a model, I have compared these ethological views with a control strategy, in which agents invariably attack others upon meeting (the 'obligate' attack strategy). The ambiguity-reducing strategy was implemented as a symmetrical rule in which an agent is more likely to attack those that are closer in rank to itself. In the 'risk-sensitive' strategy, the probability of an attack increases the lower the rank of an opponent is. Intensity of aggression is varied as follows: in intensely aggressive agents the change in dominance values that results from each interaction is increased by a scaling factor (i.e. StepDom) that is higher than in mildly aggressive agents.

The models show a suite of emergent effects: a dominance hierarchy and a social–spatial structure (with dominants in the centre, subordinates at the periphery) develop and mutually reinforce each other. These processes are accompanied by an automatic reduction of the frequency of interaction. Remarkably, it appears that frequency of aggression decreases in all three attack strategies, at least when groups are cohesive and the intensity of aggression is sufficiently high (Hemelrijk, 1999a, 2000b).

For the ambiguity-reducing strategy, this reduction of aggression is a direct consequence but for the other two strategies (namely, the obligatory and the risk-sensitive strategies) it is an unforeseen effect (Fig. 5.4). It develops because a steep hierarchy develops at a high intensity of aggression (by the strong impact each interaction has on the rank of both partners) and this automatically implies that some agents become permanent losers and therefore, fleeing repeatedly, move

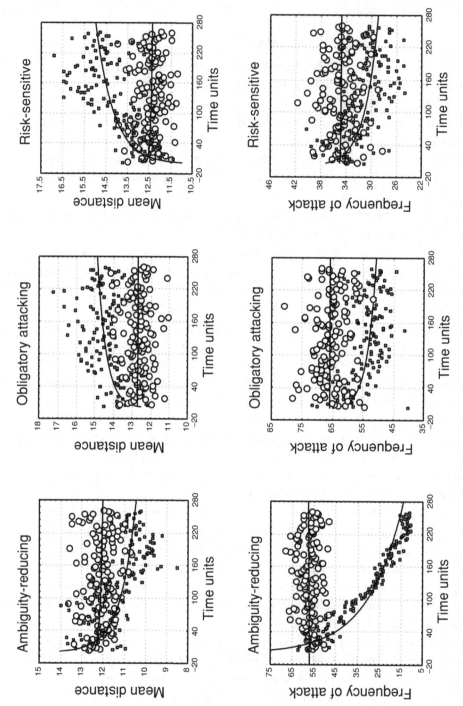

Figure 5.4 Development of mean distance (top half) and frequency of aggressive interactions (lower half) among agents for different attack strategies and intensities of aggression (logarithmic line fitting). Circles represent StepDom values of 0.1, squares values of 1.0.

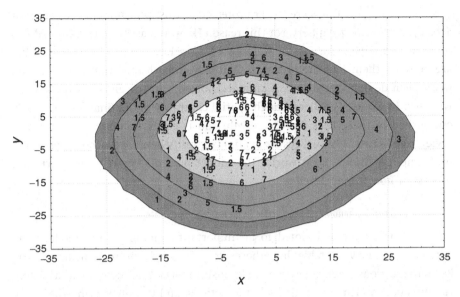

Figure 5.5 Visualisation of the social–spatial structure during the last 60 time-steps of a run. Shown are the positions of eight agents every other time-step. Numbers indicate relative rank (from 1 to 8). Surface contours are isoclines of identical mean rank and were obtained by using a cubic spline smoothing procedure. Darker shading indicates lower mean rank. StepDom 1.0 indicates high intensity of aggression.

away further and further from others. The increased distance among agents, in its turn, results in a decrease of the frequency of encounter and hence, of aggression. Thus, from the model we learn that such a reduction arises automatically as a property of the system and in the absence of any internal mechanism to reduce the frequency of attack. This suggests a test for the real world: it should be studied whether the development of the dominance hierarchy is accompanied not only by a reduction of aggression but also by an increase in mutual distances.

Spatial centrality of dominants

When behaving according to the ambiguity-reducing strategy, agents chase away those that are close in rank and therefore end up near rank-distant group members as the hierarchy differentiates. In the other two strategies, however, a spatial structure with dominants in the centre develops but this occurs only at a relatively high intensity of aggression and in relatively cohesive groups (Hemelrijk, 1999a, b, 2000b) (Fig. 5.5).

The emergence of such a spatial structure is particularly interesting because Hamilton's influential 'selfish herd' theory (Hamilton, 1971) supposes that it arises because individuals are better protected against predators in the centre of a group than at the periphery. For this reason Hamilton assumes that individuals evolved a 'centripetal instinct', a preference for the location in which conspecifics are between them and the predator. Centre-oriented locomotion has, however, never been demonstrated in real animals, not even in the elegant experiments with fish by Krause (1993), although spatial centrality of dominants was clearly established in these tests (Krause, 1994b) and is general among animals (for a review, see Krause, 1994a). Because spatial centrality develops without positional preference in the artificial world, the model presents us with an alternative process of how it may develop.

Emergent phenomena as specific hypotheses for primates

This section is devoted to an important function of the models: the derivation of new, testable hypotheses for the study of real primates. The behavioural consequences of the risk-sensitive attack strategy bear a strong resemblance to primate dominance interactions, and by only varying the intensity of aggression a remarkable correspondence emerges between patterns in the artificial worlds and those observed in the social behaviour of so-called 'egalitarian' and 'despotic' macaque species. Therefore, the understanding of the way in which these patterns emerge in the models provides a parsimonious hypothesis for the evolution of these dominance styles in macaques.

In primates and in some other species, however, individuals are able to recognise the identity of others and to memorise personal experiences with them (Barnard and Burk, 1979). In the artificial world, agents that perceive dominance of others directly are called 'Perceivers' and the others 'Estimators' (Hemelrijk, 2000b).

The dominance hierarchy and therefore the social–spatial structure among Perceivers is stronger than among Estimators. This is a consequence of the variation of experiences Estimators have with certain others (as is reflected in their memorised dominance values of the other group members). Because the dominance hierarchy and the social–spatial structure of Estimators is founded on the average conception of each agent about a certain group member, the ensuing difference of opinions about each other weakens the formation of the dominance hierarchy and the development of social–spatial structure. Also, Estimators may have triangular relationship (in which A dominates B, B dominates C, but C defies A), whereas Perceivers cannot, because they always perceive the rank of a particular group member in exactly the same way. In the remainder of this section I will deal only with Perceivers, because their behaviour gives rise to clearer patterns and because direct rank perception is probably at work in most animal species that perform dominance interactions.

Based on the assumption that spatial structure influences via proximity sociopositive behaviour, hypotheses are developed for affiliation patterns among real primates. Furthermore, in DomWorld inter-sexual dominance relations appear to vary with intensity of aggression; whether this holds for real primates, too, should be tested in a comparative study between egalitarian and despotic macaques. Since inter-sexual dominance may influence sexual behaviour, this phenomenon is used to generate hypotheses for the differences in sexual behaviour (i.e. in male mounting and female choice) between both types of macaque species. Next, varying the cohesion of grouping results in phenomena that lead to an alternative explanation of the causes of female dominance in pygmy chimpanzees. Finally, social attraction between the artificial sexes results in an increase of female dominance. This phenomenon may be used as an alternative for the supposed exchange of male tolerance offered to females for mating.

Degree of despotism in macaques

Dominance is supposed to be associated with benefits such as priority of access to mates, food and safe spatial locations. In this respect, Vehrencamp (1983) distinguishes between 'despotic' and 'egalitarian' species. In the former, benefits are strongly biased towards higher-ranking individuals, while in the latter access to resources is more equally distributed. Now, the terms despotic and egalitarian are generally used to classify social systems of many animal species (such as insects, birds and primates). Because it is difficult to estimate how benefits are distributed over group members, the gradient of the hierarchy is the characteristic used to distinguish egalitarian and despotic primates. However, egalitarian and despotic species vary in many other traits. In the majority of primatological studies, such as for instance those by van Schaik (1989), comparisons between egalitarian and despotic primate species are made within the framework of optimisation of single traits by natural selection. In contrast, Thierry (1985a) suggests that the numerous behavioural differences between egalitarian and despotic macaques can be traced back simply to internal differences in intensity of aggression and degree of nepotism (i.e. support of kin). In the present model we present an even simpler hypothesis, namely that only a difference in intensity of aggression is needed to understand the origination of both types of societies. Here we compare results of a world inhabited by 'Mild' agents (with a low intensity of aggression, represented by a low StepDom value) with one containing 'Fierce' agents (i.e. a high StepDom value).

Thierry argues that (compared to egalitarian macaques) despotic species are characterised by a lower frequency of counter-attack, because of the risk posed by their more intense form of aggression. The same is found for Fierce agents

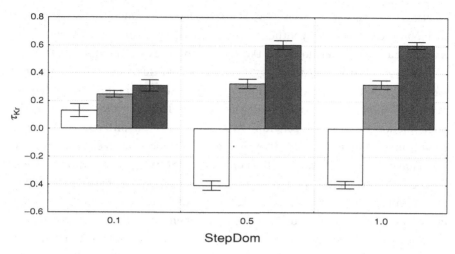

Figure 5.6 Symmetry of attack in three attack systems for varying intensities of aggression (mean $\tau_{Kr} \pm$ SE) White bars, risk-sensitive attack; shaded bars, obligate attack; hatched bars, ambiguity-reducing attack system.

compared to Mild agents, at least when they behave according to the risk-sensitive attack strategy (Hemelrijk, 1999b) (Fig. 5.6). Furthermore, Fierce virtual agents show a lower degree of group cohesiveness, a lower frequency of attack and more rank-correlated behaviour than Mild agents. All these properties resemble the differences found between despotic and egalitarian macaques (de Waal and Luttrell, 1989; Thierry, 1985a,b).

In short, the model makes clear how by changing a single parameter representing the intensity of aggression, one may switch from an egalitarian to a despotic society. Also, in the real world natural selection may accordingly have operated simply on intensity of aggression. If under certain conditions of distribution and abundance of food animals benefit from a higher intensity of aggression, then a society of individuals displaying the complete set of traits that characterise the despotic dominance style may actually evolve as a consequence of a mutation in one single trait only.

Patterns of grooming behaviour

Spatial centrality of dominants occurs in a number of primate species, particularly those that are characterised by a steep hierarchy (Itani, 1954). A similar relationship is found in the artificial worlds (among Fierce virtual agents spatial centrality of dominants is greater than among Mild agents) and this provides us with a parsimonious hypothesis for the grooming patterns among female monkeys described by Seyfarth (1977) (see Hemelrijk, 1996b). Seyfarth has traced two grooming patterns: (a) high-ranking individuals receive more grooming than others, and (b) most grooming takes place between individuals that are adjacent in rank. Seyfarth believes that two principles underlie these phenomena: (a) higher-ranking females are more attractive to groom, because potentially more benefits can be gained from them in exchange, and (b) access to preferred (i.e. higher-ranking) grooming partners is restricted by competition. Consequently, in the end each female grooms most frequently close-ranking partners and is groomed herself most often by the female ranking just below her.

Now consider what happens in the world of artificial primates. From the foregoing we know that competition leads to spatial centrality of dominants. If individuals groom others in proportion to their encounter rate, this spatial arrangement determines – through proximity – the grooming pattern at a group level. Consequently, individuals groom more often those that are nearby in rank. The same process, moreover, also explains why dominants are groomed more often than subordinates: because they are more often in the centre, dominants simply meet others more frequently. Note that this is a simpler explanation than Seyfarth's, because it does not require assumptions about exchanges for future social benefits. Besides, individuals obviously do not need to discern the relative rank of group members in order to groom higher-ranking partners more often than others, as is supposed by Seyfarth (1981). To establish the relevance of this idea for real primates, it should be tested whether the patterns of grooming as described by Seyfarth occur particularly in groups with central dominants and not in those with a weak spatial structure.

Inter-sexual dominance relationships among macaques

The close agreement with the dominance styles of macaques inspired further use of the model for developing hypotheses about male–female dominance relationships among these monkeys (Hemelrijk, 1999b). There is a dire need for such hypotheses, because – remarkably– inter-sexual relationships are largely ignored in primate studies other than those of Madagascar lemurs. For the sake of simplicity, the sexes in the artificial agents are only distinguished in terms of the inferior fighting capacity of females (i.e. the StepDom value of VirtualFemales is lower than that of VirtualMales and VirtualFemales start with a lower dominance value than VirtualMales). The sexes are distinguished for both Fierce and Mild species of agents, so there are Virtual(fierce)Males and Virtual(mild)Males and Females. Surprisingly, Virtual(fierce)Males are less dominant over VirtualFemales than Virtual(mild)Males are. This is due to the stronger hierarchical differentiation of the Fierce agents, which causes both sexes to overlap in rank more than among Mild agents (Fig. 5.7). Similarly in despotic macaques, adolescent males have greater difficulty in outranking adult females

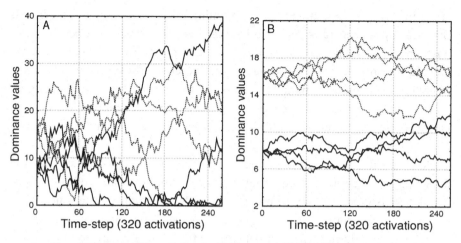

Figure 5.7 Rank differentiation in (A) Fierce and (B) Mild Virtual Species. Dotted lines, VirtualMales; solid lines, VirtualFemales.

than in egalitarian species (Thierry, 1990). Thierry explains this as a consequence of the supposed fact that cooperation to suppress males is stronger among females of despotic than of egalitarian macaques. Because of the associated benefits, van Schaik (1989) has argued that coalitions are especially advantageous for females of despotic species. Clearly, compared to the model-generated hypothesis, the views of Thierry and van Schaik are based on assumptions that are not strictly necessary for the explanation of the behaviour.

Differences in male dominance over females may affect sexual behaviour. In their study of male bonnet macaques Rosenblum and Nadler (1971) discovered an ontogenetical fact: adult males ejaculate after a single mount, whereas young males need several mounts. The authors suggest that this has to do with incomplete dominance over females and that the degree of female dominance over males may also explain similar differences in sexual behaviour at the species level. Linking these observations to the patterns of female dominance found among the artificial agents we would expect males of despotic species to enjoy less relaxed matings than males of egalitarian species do. Analogous observations have indeed been reported by Caldecott (1986): despotic male macaques mount females several times before reaching ejaculation whereas egalitarian males are single-mounters. He explains this difference using a complex argument about the evolution of adaptive differences in female choice between the two types of macaque species. The explanation derived from the model, however, is more simple: the differences in sexual behaviour between egalitarian and despotic macaques may be a consequence of the difference in male dominance over females due to different intensities of aggression, and, therefore, no specific adaptive explanation is needed.

Female dominance over males in two species of chimpanzees

Males of most primate species are bigger and stronger than females and, therefore, it is common usage to consider males to be dominant over females. Whereas indeed this is true for common chimpanzees, there is the remarkable fact that among pygmy chimpanzees certain females are frequently dominant over (some) males (Stanford, 1998). Traditionally, this is explained by suggesting that female pygmy chimpanzees have a stronger tendency to form large coalitions to suppress single males (Parish, 1994) than females of common chimpanzees. This explanation maintains the accepted image of the 'weak' female, because female dominance is not attributed to individual power, but to collective strength.

However, the degree of female dominance is not the only difference between the two chimpanzee species: pygmy chimpanzees also live in much more cohesive groups than common chimpanzees (C. K. Hemelrijk and A. Dübendorfer, unpubl. data). The study of DomWorld in which we vary the degree of cohesiveness shows that dominance differentiation is particularly marked in dense groups (Hemelrijk, 1999a) and that greater differentiation accompanies greater female dominance. Thus, female dominance over males may be a side effect of greater cohesiveness. Thus, if in real apes cohesiveness affects female dominance over males in a similar way, females in dense groups are expected to dominate males more than in loose groups. This could solve the puzzling question of the strong female dominance among pygmy chimpanzees.

Male 'tolerance' during sexual attraction

In primates, females develop a pink swelling during the period in which they can be fertilised, and during this period males are observed to allow females priority of access to food (e.g. see Goodall, 1986). This is regarded as an adaptive exchange of favours, namely priority of access to food for females in exchange for copulation for males (Tutin, 1980; Stanford, 1996). However, as mentioned above, evidence for such exchange in terms of the number of offspring is very limited, if existing at all (Hemelrijk et al., 1999). Although males do not seem to profit from it, they are more tolerant towards females during tumescence (Yerkes, 1939, 1940) and this asks for an explanation.

In primates, as in many other animal species, males are the ones who actively maintain proximity to females when females are in their sexually attractive, fertile period (see Hill, 1987). This sexual asymmetry is understandable, because males can fertilise many females, whereas females get fertilised only once per reproductive period. We used DomWorld to study whether such increased male interest in females changes inter-sexual relationships automatically in such a

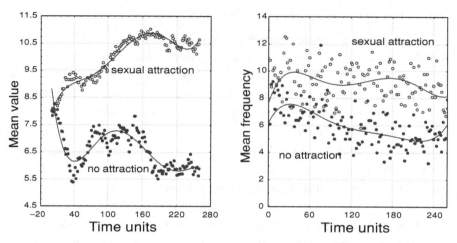

Figure 5.8 (A) Mean female dominance and (B) mean male 'tolerance' (i.e. non-aggressive proximity) to females over time. (Logarithmic line fitting).

way as to seem to increase male 'tolerance' (Hemelrijk, 2000a). Upon implementing such 'sexual attraction' of males to females as preferential male orientation towards females rather than towards males, it appears that this indeed increases female dominance over males! This arises due to the inbuilt mechanism that unexpected victories and defeats cause a greater change in the dominance values of both opponents than expected outcomes do, in combination with the higher frequency of interaction between the sexes. As a consequence of their increased dominance, females display aggression more often to males and males display it less often to females (Fig. 5.8). This looks like an increase in male 'tolerance' of females, but instead of male 'tolerance', a better name for it is male 'respectful timidity' and obviously, this is not a manipulative strategy!

Female dominance over males increases, however, only in despotic artificial societies, but not in egalitarian ones. This comes about because artificial egalitarian females are too subordinate to males to have any possibility of defeating them by accident even if males are attracted to them (Hemelrijk, 2002a). It is of interest to study whether also among real primates female dominance increases more during sexual attraction in despotic than in egalitarian societies (for a similar degree of sexual dimorphism).

Discussion and conclusion

Although individual traits (such as grooming, food sharing and support in fights) may independently have been shaped by natural selection as is usually implicitly assumed, this is probably not always the case. Certain genetic differences between species may automatically imply a large number of side effects. It is not easy to imagine how and when side effects arise, and here individual-based models, such as DomWorld, may be of help. For instance, increasing intensity of aggression in DomWorld has many consequences; it leads to a steeper hierarchy, reduced bidirectionality of aggression, a reduction of the frequency of aggression, an increase of the average distance among individuals, and spatial structure, etc.

The results mentioned here not only bear a strong resemblance to primate societies (particularly of egalitarian and despotic macaques), but also to the behaviour of fish as described in a selection experiment on the speed of growth in a study by Ruzzante and Doyle (1991, 1993). In one of their experiments fish had to get food from clumped sources, which leads to intense competition. After two generations of selection three effects were recorded: an increase in the speed of growth was accompanied by a decrease in intensity of aggression, and an increase in density of schooling and in social tolerance. The negative relation between speed of growth and aggressiveness is thought to be due to the limitation of the energy that is available. The authors explain the connection between aggression and the rest of the social behaviour, by the use of a so-called 'threshold hypothesis' for intensity of aggression: selection towards fast growth under intense food competition results in a high threshold for aggression (i.e. a reduced intensity of aggression) and this threshold also genetically influences the other two acts of social behaviour, namely cohesion and social tolerance. As regards the social behaviour observed, these findings resemble those found in DomWorld, but in DomWorld only thing that is changed 'genetically' is the intensity of aggression, and all other changes of social behaviour simply result as side effects. This presents a parsimonious alternative for the explanation of the findings in the selection experiment by Ruzzante and Doyle.

Such a view that behavioural traits are interconnected and that changes in one trait influence other traits corresponds with multi-level selection theories. For instance, in the case of the evolution of a despotic society of macaques phylogenetic studies suggest that the common ancestor of macaques was relatively egalitarian (Matsumura, 1999; Thierry et al., 2000). If certain populations of the common ancestor suffered food shortage, individuals may have benefited from a higher intensity of aggression. In such a case, as a consequence of one single adaptation only (higher intensity of aggression), a society of individuals evolves that displays the complete set of traits that characterise the despotic dominance style. Further, groups that are more strongly despotic may survive longer under food shortage, as is shown by studies of social spiders, in which groups (not individuals) of different degrees of despotism are compared. This happens because by claiming much more food than others, a few dominant individuals will get

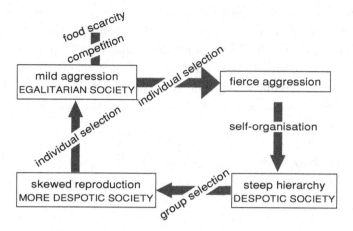

Figure 5.9 Hypothetical transitions between egalitarian and despotic societies.

enough to reproduce. In a more egalitarian society, however, the equal division of food will allow nobody to get enough to reproduce (social spiders: Ulbrich *et al.*, 1996). In such a way, despotic societies may have evolved from a combination of individual selection, self-organisation and selection at the level of the group and this may hold also for primate societies (Hemelrijk, 2002b).

Another interesting point is what happens when selection operates in the opposite direction, that is if we start from a despotic society and the availability of food increases. We may imagine how under conditions of markedly increased food quantities, all groups survive independently of their degree of despotism and thus, group selection is weakened. Further, competition within a group is reduced also, and therefore, milder animals that waste less energy in intense aggression may increase in number and thus reduce the intensity of aggression in the entire society. Consequently, no social spatial structuring takes place and what remains is a society with a weak hierarchy, a society that is egalitarian (Fig. 5.9). Thus more processes may be involved when we switch from a despotic system to an egalitarian one than when we switch the other way round.

In summary, in traditional approaches selection is supposed to operate on a single trait at the level of the individual and therefore, single traits are studied empirically. In line with multiple-level selection theory, we may, however, also imagine that selection operates at many levels, including the emergent pattern (such as the spatial structure and the gradient of the hierarchy) and the group. Under such a view, in our empirical studies, we need to investigate several traits simultaneously and we need to extend models of emergent social behaviour to an evolutionary time scale.

Acknowledgements

Work described in this paper has been partly supported by grants from the Kommission zur Foerderung des akademischen nachwuchses der Universitaet Zuerich and the Marie-Heim Voegtlin Foundation. I would like to thank Rolf Pfeifer, Bob Martin and Franjo Weissing for support.

References

Axelrod, R. and Hamilton, W. D. (1981). The evolution of cooperation. *Science* **211**, 1390–1396.

Barnard, C. J. and Burk, T. E. (1979). Dominance hierarchies and the evolution of 'individual recognition'. *J. Theoret. Biol.* **81**, 65–73.

Bernstein, I. S. and Gordon, T. P. (1980). The social component of dominance relationships in rhesus monkeys (*Macaca mulatta*). *Anim. Behav.* **28**, 1033–1039.

Bonabeau, E., Theraulaz, G. and Deneubourg, J.-L. (1996). Mathematical models of self-organizing hierarchies in animal societies. *Bull. Math. Biol.* **58**, 661–717.

Butovskaya, M., Kozintsev, A. and Welker, C. (1995). Grooming and social rank by birth: the case of *Macaca fascicularis*. *Folia Primatol.* **65**, 30–33.

Byrne, R. W. and Whiten, A. (1988). *Machiavellian Intelligence: Social Expertise and the Evolution of Intellect in Monkeys, Apes, and Humans*. Oxford: Clarendon Press.

Caldecott, J. O. (1986). Mating patterns, societies and ecogeography of macaques. *Anim. Behav.* **34**, 208–220.

Constable, J. L., Ashley, M. V., Goodall, J. and Pusey, A. E. (2001). Noninvasive paternity assignment in Gombe chimpanzees. *Mol. Ecol.* **10**, 1279–1300.

Darwin, C. (1871). *The Descent of Man and Selection in Relation to Sex*. London: John Murray.

Datta, S. B. and Beauchamp, G. (1991). Effects of group demography on dominance relationships among female primates. I. Mother–daughter and sister–sister relations. *Am. Naturalist* **138**, 201–226.

de Waal, F. B. M. (1978). Exploitative and familiarity dependent support strategies in a colony of semi-free living chimpanzees. *Behaviour* **66**, 268–312.

de Waal, F. B. M. and Luttrell, L. M. (1989). Towards a comparative socioecology of the genus *Macaca*: different dominance styles in rhesus and stumptail monkeys. *Am. J. Primatol.* **19**, 83–109.

de Waal, F. B. M. and van Hooff, J. A. R. A. M. (1981). Side-directed communication and agonistic interactions in chimpanzees. *Behaviour* **77**, 164–198.

Dugatkin, L. A., Alfieri, M. S. and Moore, J. A. (1994). Can dominance hierarchies be replicated? Form–re-form experiments using cockroach (*Nauphoeta cinerea*). *Ethology* **97**, 94–102.

Ellis, L. (1994). Reproductive and interpersonal aspects of dominance and status. In *Social Stratification and Socioeconomic Inequality*, ed. L. Ellis. Westport, CT: Greenwood, pp. 145–163.

Furuichi, T. (1985). Inter-male associations in a wild Japanese macaque troop on Yakushima island, Japan. *Primates* **26**, 219–237.

Goldberg, T. L. and Wrangham, R. W. (1997). Genetic correlates of social behaviour in wild chimpanzees: evidence from mitochondrial DNA. *Anim. Behav.* **54**, 559–570.

Goodall, J. (1986). *The Chimpanzees of Gombe: Patterns of Behaviour*. Cambridge, MA: Harvard University Press.

Guhl, A. M. (1968). Social inertia and social stability in chickens. *Anim. Behav.* **16**, 219–232.

Hamilton, W. D. (1964). The genetical evolution of social behaviour. I. *J. Theoret. Biol.* **7**, 1–16.

(1971). Geometry for the selfish herd. *J. Theoret. Biol.* **31**, 295–311.

Hamilton, W. J. and Bulger, J. (1992). Facultative expression of behavioral differences between one-male and multimale savanna baboon groups. *Am. J. Primatol.* **28**, 61–71.

Hemelrijk, C. K. (1990a). A matrix partial correlation test used in investigations of reciprocity and other social interaction patterns at a group level. *J. Theoret. Biol.* **143**, 405–420.

(1990b). Models of, and tests for, reciprocity, unidirectional and other social interaction patterns at a group level. *Anim. Behav.* **39**, 1013–1029.

(1996a). Dominance interactions, spatial dynamics and emergent reciprocity in a virtual world. In *Proc. 4th Int. Conf. Simulation of Adaptive Behavior*, pp. 545–552.

(1996b). Reciprocation in apes: from complex cognition to self-structuring. In *Great Ape Societies*, ed. W. C. McGrew, L. F. Marchant and T. Nishida. Cambridge: Cambridge University Press, pp. 185–195.

(1997). Cooperation without genes, games or cognition. In *Proc. 4th Europ. Conf. Artificial Life*, pp. 511–520.

(1999a). Effects of cohesiveness on intersexual dominance relationships and spatial structure among group-living virtual entities. In *Proc. 5th Europ. Conf. Artificial Life*, pp. 524–534.

(1999b). An individual-oriented model on the emergence of despotic and egalitarian societies. *Proc. Roy. Soc. London B* **266**, 361–369.

(2000a). Sexual attraction and inter-sexual dominance. In *Proc. 2nd Int. Workshop on Multi Agent Based Simulation*, Boston, MA, July, 2000, pp. 167–180.

(2000b). Towards the integration of social dominance and spatial structure. *Anim. Behav.* **59**, 1035–1048.

(2002a). Despotic societies, sexual attraction and the emergence of male 'tolerance': an agent-based model. *Behaviour* **139**, 729–747.

(2002b). Self-organisation and natural selection in the evolution of complex despotic societies. *Biol. Bull.* **202**, 283–289.

Hemelrijk, C. K. and Ek, A. (1991). Reciprocity and interchange of grooming and 'support' in captive chimpanzees. *Anim. Behav.* **41**, 923–935.

Hemelrijk, C. K. and Luteijn, M. (1998). Philopatry, male presence and grooming reciprocation among female primates: a comparative perspective. *Behav. Ecol. Sociobiol.* **42**, 207–215.

Hemelrijk, C. K., Klomberg, T. J. M., Nooitgedagt, J. H. and van Hooff, J. A. R. A. M. (1991). Side-directed behaviour and recruitment of support in captive chimpanzees. *Behaviour* **118**, 89–102.

Hemelrijk, C. K., van Laere, G. J. and van Hooff, J. A. R. A. M. (1992). Sexual exchange relationships in captive chimpanzees? *Behav. Ecol. Sociobiol.* **30**, 269–275.

Hemelrijk, C. K., Meier, C. M. and Martin, R. D. (1999). 'Friendship' for fitness in chimpanzees? *Anim. Behav.* **58**, 1223–1229.

Hill, D. (1987). Social relationships between adult male and female rhesus macaques. I. Sexual consortships. *Primates* **28**, 439–456.

Hinde, R. A. (1982). *Ethology*. New York: Oxford University Press.

Hogeweg, P. (1988). MIRROR beyond MIRROR, Puddles of LIFE. In *Artificial Life: SFI Studies in the Sciences of Complexity*, ed. C. Langton. Redwood City, CA: Addison-Wesley, pp. 297–316.

Hogeweg, P. and Hesper, B. (1983). The ontogeny of interaction structure in bumble bee colonies: a MIRROR model. *Behav. Ecol. Sociobiol.* **12**, 271–283.

(1985). Socioinformatic processes: MIRROR modelling methodology. *J. Theoret. Biol.* **113**, 311–330.

Itani, J. (1954). *The Monkeys of Mount Takasaki*. Tokyo: Kobunsha.

Judson, O. P. (1994). The rise of the individual-based model in ecology. *Trends Ecol. Evol.* **9**, 9–14.

Jurke, M. H., Pryce, C. R., Hug-Hodel, A. and Döbeli, M. (1995). An investigation into the socioendocrinology of infant care and postpartum fertility in Goeldi's monkey (*Callimico goeldii*). *Int. J. Primatol.* **16**, 453–474.

Krause, J. (1993). The effect of 'Schreckstoff' on the shoaling behaviour of the minnow: a test of Hamilton's selfish herd theory. *Anim. Behav.* **45**, 1019–1024.

(1994a). Differential fitness returns in relation to spatial position in groups. *Biol. Rev.* **69**, 187–206.

(1994b). The influence of food competition and predation risk on size-assortative shoaling in juvenile chub (*Leuciscus cephalus*). *Ethology* **96**, 105–116.

Kummer, H. (1974). *Rules of Dyad and Group Formation among Captive Baboons* (Theropithecus gelada). Basel: S. Karger.

Martin, R. D. (1992). Female cycles in relation to paternity in primate societies. In *Paternity in Primates: Genetic Tests and Theories*, ed. R. D. Martin, A. F. Dixson and E. J. Wickings. Basel: S. Karger, pp. 238–274.

Matsumura, S. (1999). The evolution of 'Egalitarian' and 'Despotic' social systems among macaques. *Primates* **40**, 23–31.

Mazur, A. (1985). A biosocial model of status in face-to face primate groups. *Social Forces* **64**, 377–402.

Meier, C., Hemelrijk, C. K. and Martin, R. D. (2000). Paternity determination, genetic characterization and social correlates in a captive group of chimpanzees (*Pan troglodytes*). *Primates* **41**, 175–183.

Menard, N., Scheffrahn, W., Vallet, D., Zidane, C. and Reber, C. (1992). Application of blood protein electrophoresis and DNA fingerprinting to the analysis of paternity and social characteristics of wild Barbary macaques. In *Paternity in*

Primates: Genetic Tests and Theories, ed. R. D. Martin, A. F. Dixson and E. J. Wickings. Basel: S. Karger, pp. 155–174.

Merriwether, D. A., Mitani, J. and Zhang, C. (2000). Mitochondrial DNA variation and male affiliation, and cooperation in wild chimpanzees. *Am. J. Phys. Anthropol.* **30**, 228.

Milinski, M. (1987). Tit for tat and the evolution of cooperation in sticklebacks. *Nature* **325**, 433–435.

Mitani, J. C., Watts, D. P., Pepper, J. W. and Merriwether, D. A. (2002). Demographic and social constraints on male chimpanzee behaviour. *Anim. Behav.* **64**, 727–737.

Morin, P. A. (1993). Reproductive strategies in chimpanzees. *Ybk Phys. Anthropol.* **36**, 179–212.

Pagel, M. and Dawkins, M. S. (1997). Peck orders and group size in laying hens: 'future contracts' for non-aggression. *Behav. Processes* **40**, 13–25.

Parish, A. R. (1994). Sex and food control in the 'uncommon chimpanzee': how bonobo females overcome a phylogenetic legacy of male dominance. *Ethol. Sociobiol.* **15**, 157–179.

Paul, A., Kuester, J. and Arnemann, J. (1992). DNA fingerprinting reveals that infant care by male Barbary macaques (*Macaca sylvanus*) is not investment. *Folia Primatol.* **58**, 93–98.

Pusey, A. E. and Packer, C. (1987). Dispersal and philopatry. In *Primate Societies*, ed. B. B. Smuts, D. L. Cheney, R. M. Seyfarth, R. W. Wrangham and T. T. Struhsaker, Chicago, IL: Chicago University Press, pp. 250–266.

Rosenblum, L. A. and Nadler, R. D. (1971). The ontogeny of sexual behavior in male bonnet macaques. In *Influence of Hormones on the Nervous System*, ed. D. H. Ford. Basel: S. Karger, pp. 388–400.

Ruzzante, D. E. and Doyle, R. W. (1991). Rapid behavioral changes in medaka caused by selection for competitive and noncompetitive growth. *Evolution* **45**, 1936–1946.

   (1993). Evolution of social behaviour in a resource rich, structured environment: selection experiments with medaka. *Evolution* **47**, 456–470.

Seyfarth, R. M. (1977). A model of social grooming among adult female monkeys. *J. Theoret. Biol.* **65**, 671–698.

   (1981). Do monkeys rank each other? *Behav. Brain Sci.* **4**, 447–448.

Stanford, C. B. (1996). The hunting ecology of wild chimpanzees: implications for the evolutionary ecology of Pliocene hominids. *Am. Anthropol.* **98**, 96–113.

   (1998). The social behaviour of chimpanzees and bonobos. *Curr. Anthropol.* **39**, 399–420.

Stephens, D. W., Anderson, J. P. and Benson, K. E. (1997). On the spurious occurrence of Tit for Tat in pairs of predator-approaching fish. *Anim. Behav.* **53**, 113–131.

te Boekhorst, I. J. A. and Hogeweg, P. (1994). Selfstructuring in artificial 'CHIMPS' offers new hypotheses for male grouping in chimpanzees. *Behaviour* **130**, 229–252.

Teleki, G. (1973). *The Predatory Behaviour of Wild Chimpanzees.* Lewisburg, PA: Bucknell University Press.

Thierry, B. (1985a). Patterns of agonistic interactions in three species of macaque (*Macaca mulatta, M. fascicularis, M. tonkeana*). *Aggress. Behav.* **11**, 223–233.

(1985b). Social development in three species of macaque (*Macaca mulatta, M. fascicularis, M. tonkeana*). *Behav. Processes* **11**, 89–95.

(1990). Feedback loop between kinship and dominance: the macaque model. *J. Theoret. Biol.* **145**, 511–521.

Thierry, B., Iwaniuk, A. N. and Pellis, S. M. (2000). The influence of phylogeny on the social behaviour of macaques (Primates: Cercopithecidae, genus *Macaca*). *Ethology* **106**, 713–728.

Trivers, R. L. (1971). The evolution of reciprocal altruism. *Q. Rev. Biol.* **46**, 35–57.

Tutin, C. E. G. (1980). Reproductive behaviour of wild chimpanzees in the Gombe National Park. *J. Reprod. Fertil.* Suppl. **28**, 43–57.

Ulbrich, K., Henschel, J. R., Jeltsch, F. and Wissel, C. (1996). Modelling individual variability in a social spider colony (*Stegodyphus dumicola*: Eresidae) in relation to food abundance and its allocation. In *Proc. 13th Int. Cong. Arachnology*, pp. 661–670.

van Schaik, C. P. (1989). The ecology of social relationships amongst female primates. In *Comparative Socioecology: The Behavioural Ecology of Humans and Other Mammals*, ed. V. Standen and G. R. A. Foley. Oxford: Blackwell, Scientific Publications, pp. 195–218.

Vehrencamp, S. L. (1983). A model for the evolution of despotic versus egalitarian societies. *Anim. Behav.* **31**, 667–682.

Wallis, J. (1997). A survey of reproductive parameters in the free-ranging chimpanzees in Gombe National park. *J. Reprod. Fertil.* **109**, 297–307.

Whiten, A. and Byrne, R. W. (1986). The St. Andrews catalogue of tactical deception on primates. *St. Andrews Psychological Report* **10**.

(1997). *Machiavellian Intelligence*, vol. 2, *Extensions and Evaluations*. Cambridge: Cambridge University Press.

Wrangham, R. W. (1980). An ecological model of female-bonded primate groups. *Behaviour* **75**, 262–300.

Yerkes, R. M. (1939). Social dominance and sexual status in chimpanzees. *Q. Rev. Biol.* **14**, 115–136.

(1940). Social behavior of chimpanzees: dominance between mates in relation to sexual status. *J. Comp. Psychol.* **30**, 147–186.

6

Order and noise in primate societies

BERNARD THIERRY

Centre d'Ecologie, Physiologie et Ethologie, CNRS, Strasbourg

As students of animal societies, we claim we observe levels of organi-sation, networks of relationships, mating systems and demographic structures. We identify classes, matrilines and hierarchies. We consider things like parental investment, nepotistic patterns or dominance strategies. We try to explain the patterning of these behavioural characters by looking for their fitness. Hidden in such an endeavour is a common assumption among scientists: the world and its objects exist independently of any observer; scientists have to discover these objects. Such a stance is known as metaphysical realism (Putnam, 1981). In bio-logy, this implies that we assume natural selection to act upon characters we observe. But 'How would we know if social organizations were *not* adaptive?' (Rowell, 1979). Even if we are not acquainted with philosophical thinking, we should be warned against the appearance fallacy. We are aware that the brain reconstructs reality from electrical signals transmitted by the sensorial organs. We do not perceive social organisations per se. As Ashby (1962) puts it, the organ-isation exists in part in the eye of the beholder. What is seen may be named *sociodemographic forms*, which means, sets of individuals that are distributed and behave in a structured manner (Thierry, 1994). Sociodemographic forms repre-sent the phenomenon, the visible aspect of social organisations. If we attempt to reduce them to adaptive strategies, this may amount to attributing an adaptive function to reified structures, in other words to endowing appearances with a fitness (Thierry, 1997).

Separating selected phenomena from unselected ones should be a main task of evolutionists (Williams, 1966). The question is how to recognise the features on

Self-Organisation and Evolution of Social Systems, ed. Charlotte K. Hemelrijk.
Published by Cambridge University Press. © Cambridge University Press 2005.

which evolution can act. In complex systems, single causes may produce multiple effects. Whereas some characters have been shaped by natural selection, others are secondary consequences of the former (Williams, 1966; Gould and Lewontin, 1979). Most evolutionists recognise the existence of side effects and incidental by-products in biological organisations (Pigliucci and Kaplan, 2000). Yet this agreement only holds at superficial theoretical levels. Clashes occur when we come to concrete examples (e.g. Alcock, 1987; Gould, 1987; Sherman, 1988; Jamieson, 1989). One side emphasises function and adaptation. It dismisses by-products as being no more than trivial appendices soon to be swept away by the selective process. It believes individual strategies to be made quasi-optimal by the selective process. The other side praises structures, epigenesis and self-organisation. It sees by-products as significant parts of the evolutionary process. It tries to grasp the emerging patterns of organisations. The dialogue between both parties is difficult because it relies more on unspoken philosophical assumptions about the relative roles of contingency and necessity in nature than upon scientific evidence.

Any form is an order, reflecting a distribution which departs from equiprobability. Something similar may be said for functional patterns, the origin of which implies the intervention of an *in-form-ative* process. Discussing the respective value of both kinds of explanations requires a fair recognition of both functional and epigenetic constraints. In what follows, I will advocate the heuristic value of the epigenetic stream in distinguishing noise and order in the social organisations of non-human primates.

Adaptive order or disorder?

In Darwinian thought, evolution consists of random variation followed by selection. Order in nature is created by the intervention of natural selection. In such classical opposition between order and chance, emphasis is put on the action of ultimate factors. This functionalist approach has proved to be an effective method of uncovering the significance of biological characters. Calculating costs and benefits helps us to recognise the factors relevant to the selection process. Making assumptions about the fitness of characters allows for the generation and testing of hypotheses. By focusing on the individual's characters and strategies, however, this approach has no way to screen patterns that have no direct function. To illustrate this point, I will choose concrete examples from primate behaviour, namely infanticide, allo-mothering and interference in mating. Immature primates undergo a long period of dependency, allowing room for the intervention of conspecifics other than the mother during the developmental process. Conspecifics' behaviours may affect the fate of offspring positively or negatively. Since the main currency of evolution is the number of descendants left by individuals, behaviours related to reproduction and the survival of immature offspring cannot be disregarded as being of secondary importance.

Male infanticide

The most extreme instance of negative intervention upon offspring is infant-killing committed by adult males. About 60 cases have been reported in the wild in the last three decades (van Schaik, 2000). According to the sexual selection hypothesis, males eliminate the unweaned offspring of rivals to interrupt mothers' lactational amenorrhoea and accelerate their return to fertility. Males would then inseminate the females and eventually increase their genetic representation in future generations (Hrdy, 1974, 1979). Infanticide generally occurs at a time of social instability. As predicted by the sexual selection hypothesis, a majority of cases of infanticide follow either the immigration of an adult male who defeats and/or ousts the previous resident male, or the rise in rank of an adult male within a group. In most cases, the male appears unrelated to the infant and, though evidence is limited, it is likely that many females return to sexual receptivity somewhat earlier than if the infants had lived (van Schaik, 2000).

Most textbooks quote infanticide by male primates as a 'staple theorem of sociobiology' (Sommer, 2000). Yet several inconsistencies have been noted with regard to the adaptive interpretation of this classic example:

(1) a majority of infants survive to male replacement or rise in rank
(2) immatures are sometimes killed though they are already weaned
(3) in seasonal breeders like lemurs (*Lemur* or *Eulemur* sp.) infanticide can hardly affect the place of the annual birth
(4) in instances of cannibalism reported in chimpanzees (*Pan troglodytes*) it is not rare that the killers may have sired the victim
(5) a number of infant-killings have been described in the context of encounters between groups or with bachelor males, in which case infanticidal males would rarely have sexual access to mothers (Bernstein, 1987; Hiraiwa-Hasegawa, 1992; Bartlett *et al.*, 1993).

Infants are most often hurt when they are clinging to the mother. Challenging males attack several individuals and redirect in particular towards the weakest individuals. Infant-killing may thus be an accidental consequence of a situation of generalised conflict (Boggess, 1979; Bartlett *et al.*, 1993). In such a perspective, infanticide is not a reproductive strategy pursued by an individual, but a by-product of male aggression, i.e. noise generated by the social organisation. Whereas a bite only wounds an adult female, it leads to the death of an infant.

Rates of infant-killing vary as a correlated response to the levels of aggression performed by adult males. The selected character is the aggressiveness of males, which allows them to succeed in conflicts and competition (Bartlett et al., 1993).

For a dozen years, male infanticide has been increasingly considered as a main selective force having shaped many features of primate social organisations. To protect their offspring, females would follow various counter-strategies: migrating to neighbouring groups, forming coalitions with other females, increasing group size, establishing bonds with protecting males, confusing paternity by multiple mating or ovulation concealment (Janson and van Schaik, 2000). Such strategies would explain why infanticide is more prevalent in single-male groups than in multi-male groups. While it may be true that the presence of several males may discourage infant-killing, this does not set it up to be a female adaptive strategy against infanticidal males. Males who are able to live with each other throughout the entire year are, by definition, more socially tolerant than males who regularly evict each other. Interspecific variations in levels of social tolerance and aggression may create spurious correlations between the rates of infanticide and the numbers of adult males in a group. It may just be that the prevalence of infanticide in non-human primates is too low to explain anything about their social relationships. This would mean that all endeavours made in that direction, in the hope of discovering order under noise, would have been a waste of time.

Most proponents of the sexual selection hypothesis consider the debate about the function of infanticide as a sterile controversy (Janson and van Schaik, 2000) whereas the minority stream, which favours the by-product hypothesis, qualifies infanticide as a 'sociobiological myth' (Schubert, 1982; Bartlett et al., 1993). A main issue relates to the mortality rates of infants. We know very little about the sources of mortality among non-human primate infants (Strier, 2000). Most reports about infanticides are case studies. This may bias the literature and lead us to overestimate infanticide rates; when a group takeover or a rise in rank has no harming consequences, nothing is published. A majority of authors contend that infant-killing remains a rare event among groups of non-human primates. One may question whether the evolutionary process can select and maintain behaviours that occur sporadically (Bartlett et al., 1993). Without strong data about the sociodemographic context, there is no way to settle the question. Each is left with his/her own beliefs, and both schools may continue to oppose each other concerning the topic.

Immatures' interference in mating

In many primate species, immature individuals approach and contact copulating partners; they direct toward them various expressions and gestures,

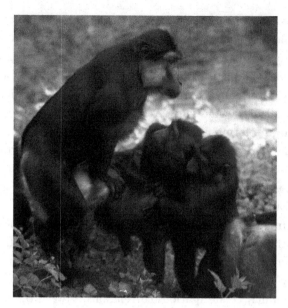

Figure 6.1 Juveniles address affiliative signals toward a mating pair of Tonkean macaques (grade 4).

either affiliative or submissive, and sometimes aggressive (Niemeyer and Anderson, 1983) (Fig. 6.1). Several explanations have been formulated with regard to the ultimate causes of such behaviours (Niemeyer and Chamove, 1983; Dixson, 1998). The protective hypothesis proposes that interference protects the mating female from possible male aggression. The reproductive potential hypothesis proposes that the immatures try to prevent the fertilisation of its mother in order to delay the birth of a rival that would monopolise the female's attention. The sentinel hypothesis suggests that the immatures aim to draw attention to the mating pair, making it likely that adult males will approach and interrupt mating. These different hypotheses have in fact received little support from empirical data. The female involved in mating is not always the mother, interference does not protect the female, and immatures' behaviours do not prevent repeated copulations between mates nor insemination of the female.

On proximate grounds, it may be noticed that immatures exhibit intense reactions to mating that involves a partner with whom they have developed strong affective ties. This suggests they are attempting to participate in the interaction or protect their social relationships (Tutin, 1979; Niemeyer and Chamove, 1983; Thierry, 1986a). In such a view, interference in mating appears as a by-product of a general psychological character aiming to protect relationships. To express it more simply, interference would be an inconsequential effect of 'jealousy', 'anxiety' or 'curiosity', psychological traits that may be adaptive in other contexts. Such a null hypothesis with regard to natural selection is however difficult to test directly.

It should be added that rates of interference vary considerably among primate species. It is common in certain species, and rare or absent in many others (Niemeyer and Chamove, 1983). No functional hypotheses so far have been able to account for such interspecific differences. It has been hypothesised that the occurrence frequency of interference depends on the level of tolerance of adult males in a species. The latter would tolerate immatures' interference in their matings only in species characterised by a relatively weak degree of dominance asymmetry among individuals (Thierry, 1986a). This hypothesis cannot be tested without extensive knowledge about social relationships in a fair sample of primate species. We need quantified comparative data to assess whether immature interference is mere disorder in the mating of adult individuals or a relevant pattern that reveals a hidden order.

Allo-mothering behaviour

In allo-mothering, the infant is handled, carried, groomed or protected by females other than the mother, mainly the youngest females. Though this behaviour usually appears as benevolent care, in some cases the infant is snatched from the mother, and in other instances handling is rough and may even harm the infant (Hrdy, 1976). A number of functionalist hypotheses have been proposed to explain infant handling. It is alternatively considered as: (1) a form of socialisation and help for the infant, (2) a learning process for the young females, (3) an assistance to the mother, or on the contrary (4) an abusive treatment intended to reduce the offspring of a rival female (Hrdy, 1976; Maestripieri, 1994). Though each of these hypotheses can account for some aspects of allo-maternal handling, none of these hypotheses can explain all kinds of handling.

A further hypothesis should be examined, namely the null hypothesis with respect to natural selection. Allo-mothering would not be adaptive, but a by-product of the social organisation. In such a view, female attraction to infants is the trait selected by the evolutionary process (Quiatt, 1979) (Fig. 6.2). It is vital in animals with extended periods of growth and development like primates. Newborns have distinctive morphological signs. It would be difficult to understand why females, who must pay considerable attention to their own offspring, would show no interest in other mothers' infants. For that to be possible, one would have to postulate that selective attachment processes occur during brief sensitive periods, which is incompatible with what we know about primates' learning abilities. These abilities are independent of context, that is, something learned in one situation can be generalised to another situation. The non-adaptive hypothesis renders understandable the various forms of allo-maternal

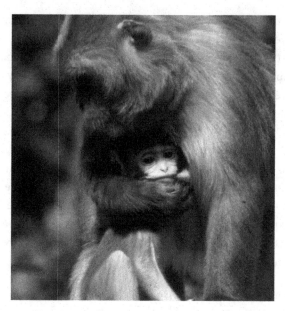

Figure 6.2 Mother performs a protective gesture over her infant in rhesus macaques (grade 1).

behaviour, whether clumsy or adroit. It parsimoniously accounts for such extreme behaviours as adoption, which saves an infant, and kidnapping, which on the contrary can bring about its death by starvation. It should be added that this hypothesis in no way forbids that allo-maternal behaviour may bring advantages for nutrition and reproduction. It can allow the mother to devote more time to food searching (Stanford, 1992) and decrease the inter-birth interval by reducing the time spent with the infant at her breast (Fairbanks, 1990).

There is an additional characteristic of allo-mothering behaviours that remains to be explained. The rates of infant handling vary widely among primate species. It is common in many colobine monkeys and some macaque species, but it is rare or limited to kin-related females in many cercopithecine monkeys and certain macaque species (McKenna, 1979; Maestripieri, 1994; Thierry, 2000). Functional hypotheses offer no explanations of why rates should differ among primate species. As for male infanticide of infants and immatures' interference in mating, we need extensive comparative data to understand the meaning of such variation.

Structural order

By focusing on individual reproducers, most evolutionary thinking points to the ordering action of natural selection. Exclusively focusing on individual strategies may be misleading, however. Any feature that is not a direct outcome of the selective process appears just as noise and disorder. The phenotype is not built only from genomic information, but also from self-organisational rules that arise through the epigenetic process. This generates structures, meaning order (Kauffman, 1993; Camazine *et al.*, 2001). Uncovering the building mechanisms requires a holistic viewpoint, which alone can account for the multiple interrelations occurring between numerous phenotypic elements. Yet the holistic enterprise is problematic. We rarely have comprehensive knowledge about complex systems and social organisations. Most people dismiss the holistic way as an impossible achievement. They instead favour the functionalist, atomistic stance, following the Cartesian principles of dividing the problem in as many sections as necessary, and progressing from the simplest to the most complex (Thierry, 1997).

As previously stated, it is not possible at present to settle the question of the function of infanticide by males, due to the current lack of demographic data. On the other hand, we can better understand the meaning of infant handling and immatures' interference in mating, by examining them in the light of the social organisations of macaques. A good record of comparative data is available in these species, providing a case in which our knowledge about the whole system is sufficient to make predictions about how the parts of the system should be.

Covariation between social patterns in macaque organisations

Among the 20 species of macaques, a dozen are fairly well known. Macaques are mainly frugivorous, semi-terrestrial primates. They form multi-male–multi-female groups, which contain both adult males and females with their offspring. Females constitute kin-bonded subgroups within their natal group while most males transfer between groups at maturation. Beyond these basic patterns of organisation, broad interspecific variation is observed within the genus with regard to aggression, conciliation, dominance and nepotism.

The degree of asymmetry in conflicts is especially variable among macaques (Thierry, 2000). In rhesus and Japanese macaques, contests are highly uni-directional: the target of aggression generally flees or submits, and severe biting is not rare. Post-conflict friendly reunions between previous opponents (i.e. reconciliations) are not frequent. The conciliatory tendencies measured among unrelated individuals consistently rated between 4% and 12% in six different groups of rhesus and Japanese macaques.

This picture departs from that observed in the Tonkean, moor and crested macaques (all species from the Sulawesi Island) where a majority of aggressive acts induce protests or counter-attacks from the targets. The intensity of aggression is low, biting is neither frequent nor injurious. Measures of conciliatory tendency yield high values: reconciliation tends to occur as much as 50% of the time among unrelated partners. Other macaque species are located intermediately between the rhesus and Japanese macaques and the Sulawesi macaques. According to aggression and reconciliation patterns, long-tailed and pig-tailed macaques are more similar to rhesus and Japanese macaques, whereas stump-tailed, Barbary and lion-tailed macaques tend toward the Sulawesi macaques.

The species-specific style of social relationships also appears to covary with the above patterns. The dominance gradient is the steepest in rhesus and Japanese macaques, the social life of which is governed by rigid hierarchies (Kawamura, 1958/65; Sade, 1972; Kurland, 1977; de Waal, 1989). Power asymmetry determines who may interact with whom. It affects how an individual chooses partners for proximity, affiliation or play, and whether the distribution of choices is skewed in favour of higher-ranking individuals. Subordinate individuals may be inhibited from approaching or contacting higher-ranking individuals because of the possibility, and subsequent cost, of attack. Females have a high preference for relatives and strong kinship bonds feature social networks.

The dominance gradient is substantially less strong in Sulawesi macaques for which status differences do not hinder contacts between group members and have little effect on grooming distribution (Thierry *et al.*, 1990, 1994; Matsumura, 1991; Petit *et al.*, 1992). Kin-bias is weak and it is not possible to characterise the social structure using proximity patterns only (Thierry *et al.*, 1990, 1994; Matsumura and Okamoto, 1997). Still other species (e.g. stump-tailed and Barbary macaques) display intermediate patterns in power asymmetry. In addition, the degree to which females prefer kin in affiliative contact, social grooming and support in conflicts is medium in the latter species (de Waal and Luttrell, 1989; Butovskaya, 1993; Aureli *et al.*, 1997).

The correlations found between reconciliation rates and the intensity and asymmetry of aggression may be explained by proximate mechanisms. Competitors' readiness to fight for resources depends on the risk incurred by doing so. If the risk of injury is high, the best tactic for the target of aggression is to avoid the opponent rather than to counter-attack. On the other hand, when targets can easily retaliate, initial aggressors risk becoming the recipients of sharp and dangerous attacks. By facilitating information exchange, conciliatory behaviours may prevent conflict and improve social relationships (Thierry, 1986b; de Waal and Luttrell, 1989). Additionally, the occurrence of conciliatory behaviours might subsequently affect aggression levels because group members are less willing to jeopardise valuable relationships. Using computerised models, it is possible to show there is a natural reinforcement between the hierarchy and the spatial distribution of animals; varying the intensity of aggression leads to a cascade

Table 6.1 *Scaling of social relationships in the genus* Macaca. *Species are ordered based on their social tolerance, which increases from the left (grade 1) to the right (grade 4), and based on their dominance gradient and kin-bias, which decreases from left to right*[a]

Grade 1	Grade 2	Grade 3	Grade 4
Rhesus macaque (*M. mulatta*)	Long-tailed macaque (*M. fascicularis*)	Lion-tailed macaque (*M. silenus*)	Tonkean macaque (*M. tonkeana*)
Japanese macaque (*M. fuscata*)	Pig-tailed macaque (*M. nemestrina*)	Barbary macaque (*M. sylvanus*)	Moor macaque (*M. maurus*)
		Stump-tailed macaque (*M. arctoides*)	Crested macaque (*M. nigra*)
		Bonnet macaque (*M. radiata*)	

[a] A number of characters vary consistently from one species to another: degree of asymmetry in conflicts, rate of conciliatory behaviours, intensity of aggression, dominance gradient, development of affiliative interactions, degree of kin preference among females, degree of mother permissiveness, amount of allo-maternal care and rate of immatures' interference in mating.

of effects that succeed in reproducing the different patterns of aggression and dominance observed in macaque relations (Hemelrijk, 1999).

Epigenetic processes

Macaque social organisations appear to belong to a finite set of possible forms. From the above behaviour patterns, macaques may be ordered along a four-grade scale going from species characterized by strict hierarchies on one side to others featured by more tolerant relationships on the other (Thierry, 2000) (Table 6.1). The scale may be used as a periodic table. It provides an operational framework that allows one to generate falsifiable hypotheses. From knowing that a species is characterised by high conciliatory rates, for instance, we may infer it should also be featured with a weak kinship bias in social relationships.

The meaning of behaviours may be examined in the light of the scale. The rates of immatures' interference in mating significantly differ between macaque species. Interferences are frequent in stump-tailed, lion-tailed and Sulawesi macaques (grades 3 and 4) (Fig. 6.1). They are rare in long-tailed macaques (grade 2), and they never occur in pig-tailed macaques (grade 2) and rhesus and Japanese macaques (grade 1) (de Benedictis, 1973; Dixson, 1977; Niemeyer and Chamove, 1983; Gore, 1986; Thierry, 1986a; Kumar, 1987; Matsumura, 1995). Such variation may be explained without resorting to any adaptive function about immatures' behaviour. If any young individual is driven to approach and interfere in the matings of adults, it will be allowed to do so only in species in

which males tolerate such disturbances. Thus, it is understandable that interference is limited or absent in the least tolerant species, in which immatures
would incur strong punishments from adult males, i.e. in grades 1 and 2.
Psychological traits like anxiety or jealousy, which are involved in the protection
of social relationships in general, would produce interference in mating as a side
effect. In such a view, the occurrence of immatures' interference is a pleiotropic
effect of an individual trait upon the social organisation (Thierry, 1997). From
the fact that bonnet macaques belong to grade 3 (Table 6.1), for instance, we
may predict that immature interference should occur in this species though it
has yet to be reported.

The same kind of thinking may be applied to the differential rates of allo-
mothering in macaques. In grades 3 and 4, infant care is frequent and most
females in a group may handle or carry them from an early age. By contrast,
the amount of infant handling by females other than the mother is limited in
grades 1 and 2, and it is in fact mostly limited to kin-related females (Thierry,
2000). Such variation is related to interspecific differences in maternal behaviour,
which appear to covary with tolerance and asymmetry in social relationships.
Except for the highest-ranking females, mothers in the first two grades are quite
protective of infants; living in a social milieu characterised by intense aggression and marked hierarchies, they frequently retrieve their infants and restrict
their interactions to relatives (Fig. 6.2). Mothers belonging to species from the
other two grades behave more confidently, they are quite permissive and allow
their offspring to move about unrestricted (Thierry, 2000). Considering the non-
adaptive hypothesis about allo-mothering within this scope allows the prediction
that the frequency of this behaviour is related to the mother's degree of protec-
tiveness and to the level of inter-individual tolerance shown in the species. This
line of reasoning may be formulated in three terms: (1) all females have strong
attraction towards infants in any species, but (2) females may express this attraction toward infants only in species in which the mother is tolerant enough to
allow allo-maternal interventions, thus (3) allo-mothering should be common in
species characterised by open relationships, and uncommon in species in which
relationships are more constrained by dominance and nepotism.

The amount of allo-mothering appears to be a direct consequence of the
mother's behaviour. All females are interested by infants but only those per-
mitted by mothers may have access to them, producing the interspecific variations we observe among macaques. Rephrasing the hypothesis in terms of epigenetic constraints may be put as follows: the generalized interest in infants is
a pleiotropic effect of maternal character; it results from a phenotypic incom-
patibility between the possession of elaborated learning abilities and a selective
attraction of females to their own offspring. It can be expressed only if social

structures are favourable, i.e. when power asymmetry is weak enough in the species for the mother to allow her companions to carry her infant. Whereas allo-mothering may be considered as noise from the point of view of natural selection, it appears from the epigenetic perspective as a peculiar product of the individual and social phenotypes of macaques. The interconnection among variables indicate that natural selection acts on self-structuring rules rather than on social patterns (see Hemelrijk, 1999).

Conclusion

The search for universal laws without concern for specific developmental and evolutionary pathways may be misleading. A behaviour such as infanticide might well be a selected trait in rodents, but this cannot be used as evidence for its adaptive value in primates (see van Schaik, 2000). If the role of individuals in evolution is stressed in an unbalanced way, behaviours become a mere expression of adaptive strategies, and sociodemographic forms appear as puzzles, the pieces of which are made of separate strategies. Acknowledging that structure and order are ascribed by the observer implies that a close examination of sociodemographic forms is necessary before resorting to selective processes.

For living beings meaning is cast upon nature by the observer and order cannot be defined in the same manner as in physics (e.g., Boltzmann, Shannon: see Atlan, 1979). The information encoded in the genes does not suffice to describe the whole phenotype. Once proteins have been fabricated, the epigenetic process starts, giving its shape to the phenotype through the enaction of local rules and multiple feedbacks. Specifying how important features of sociodemographic forms may be produced by constraints internal to organisations does not refute the role of natural selection (Camazine *et al.*, 2001). Rather, it shifts the main target of the selective process from complex patterns and strategies to individual characters and behaviours, a quite orthodox Darwinian stance by the way.

A number of patterns of macaque societies may be explained in a holistic manner. It may be expected that the role of epigenetic processes become all the more important as the distance from the level of expression of the genome increases. It is thus at the level of the social phenotype that we must expect to encounter the most powerful effects of self-organisation. Studying the links between *evolution* and *development* is a rapidly growing area of inquiry. In spite of the acknowledged importance of learning and development in animals, this field (colloquially known as 'evo/devo') is yet largely ignored in the study of social behaviour. Integrating the existence of internal rules, which arise from the epigenetic process and give rise to the structures we observe, should help to better understand their meaning and possible function.

References

Alcock, J. (1987). Ardent adaptationism. *Nat. Hist.* **96**, 4.

Ashby, W. R. (1962). Principles of the self-organising system. In *Principles of Organization*, ed. H. von Foerster and G. W. Zopf. New York: Pergamon Press, pp. 255–278.

Atlan, H. (1979). *Entre le Cristal et la Fumée*. Paris: Editions du Séuil.

Aureli, F., Das, M. and Veenema, H. C. (1997). Differential kinship effect on reconciliation in three species of macaques (*Macaca fascicularis, M. fuscata* and *M. sylvanus*). *J. Comp. Psychol.* **111**, 91–99.

Bartlett, T. Q., Sussman, R. W. and Cheverud, J. M. (1993). Infant killing in primates: a review of observed cases with specific reference to the sexual selection hypothesis. *Am. Anthropol.* **95**, 958–990.

Bernstein, I. S. (1987). The evolution of nonhuman primate social behavior. *Genetica* **73**, 99–116.

Boggess, J. (1979). Troop male membership changes and infant killing in langurs (*Presbytis entellus*). *Folia Primatol.* **32**, 65–107.

Butovskaya, M. (1993). Kinship and different dominance styles in groups of three species of the genus *Macaca* (*M. arctoides, M. mulatta, M. fascicularis*). *Folia Primatol.* **60**, 210–224.

Camazine, S., Deneubourg, J. L., Franks, N. R. *et al.* (2001). *Self-Organisation in Biological Systems*. Princeton, NJ: Princeton University Press.

de Benedictis, T. (1973). The behavior of young primates during adult copulations: observations of a *Macaca irus* colony. *Am. Anthropol.* **75**, 1469–1484.

de Waal, F. B. M. (1989). *Peacemaking among Primates*. Cambridge, MA: Harvard University Press.

de Waal, F. B. M. and Luttrell, L. M. (1989). Toward a comparative socioecology of the genus *Macaca*: different dominance styles in rhesus and stumptailed macaques. *Am. J. Primatol.* **19**, 83–109.

Dixson, A. F. (1977). Observations on the displays, menstrual cycles and sexual behaviour of the 'black ape' of Celebes (*Macaca nigra*). *J. Zool.* **182**, 63–84.

(1998). *Primate Sexuality*. Oxford: Oxford University Press.

Fairbanks, L. A. (1990). Reciprocal benefits of allomothering for female vervet monkeys. *Anim. Behav.* **40**, 553–562.

Gore, M. A. (1986). Mother–offspring conflict and interference at mother's mating in *Macaca fascicularis*. *Primates* **27**, 205–214.

Gould, S. J. (1987). Stephen Jay Gould replies. *Nat. Hist.* **96**, 4–5.

Gould, S. J. and Lewontin, R. (1979). The spandrels of San Marco and the Panglossian paradigm: a critique of the adaptationist programme. *Proc. Roy. Soc. London B* **205**, 581–598.

Hemelrijk, C. K. (1999). An individual-oriented model on the emergence of despotic and egalitarian societies. *Proc. Roy. Soc. London B* **266**, 361–369.

Hiraiwa-Hasegawa, M. (1992). Cannibalism among non-human primates. In *Cannibalism: Ecology and Evolution among Diverse Taxa*, ed. M. Elgar. Oxford: Oxford University Press, pp. 323–338.

Hrdy, S. B. (1974). Male–male competition and infanticide among the langurs (*Presbytis entellus*) of Abu, Rajasthan. *Folia Primatol.* **22**, 19–58.

  (1976). Care and exploitation of nonhuman primates by conspecifics other than the mother. *Adv. Study Behav.* **6**, 101–158.

  (1979). Infanticide among animals: a review, classification, and examination of the implications for the reproductive strategies of females. *Ethol. Sociobiol.* **1**, 13–40.

Jamieson, I. G. (1989). Levels of analysis or analyses at the same level. *Anim. Behav.* **37**, 696–697.

Janson, C. H. and van Schaik, C. P. (2000). The behavioral ecology of infanticide by males. In *Infanticide by Males and its Implications*, ed. C. P. van Schaik and C. H. Janson. Cambridge: Cambridge University Press, pp. 469–494.

Kauffman, S. S. (1993). *The Origins of Order*. Oxford: Oxford University Press.

Kawamura, S. (1958/65). Matriarchal social ranks in the Minoo-B troop: a study of the rank system of Japanese macaques. *Primates* **1**, 149–156. (In Japanese) (Translation: In *Japanese Monkeys*, ed. S. A. Altmann. Atlanta, GA: Emory University Press, pp. 105–112.)

Kumar, A. (1987). The ecology and population dynamics of the lion-tailed macaque (*Macaca silenus*) in South India. Ph.D. thesis, Cambridge University.

Kurland, J. A. (1977). *Kin Selection in the Japanese Monkey*. Basel: S. Karger.

Maestripieri, D. (1994). Social structure, infant handling, and mothering styles in group-living Old World monkeys. *Int. J. Primatol.* **15**, 531–553.

Matsumura, S. (1991). A preliminary report on the ecology and social behavior of moor macaques (*Macaca maurus*) in Sulawesi, Indonesia. *Kyoto Univ. Overseas Res. Rep. Studies in Asian Non-Human Primates* **8**, 27–41.

  (1995). Affiliative mounting interference in *Macaca maurus*. *Kyoto Univ. Overseas Res. Rep. Studies in Asian Non-Human Primates* **9**, 1–5.

Matsumura, S. and Okamoto, K. (1997). Factors affecting proximity among members of a wild group of moor macaques during, feeding, moving, and resting. *Int. J. Primatol.* **18**, 929–940.

McKenna, J. J. (1979). The evolution of allomothering among colobine monkeys: function and opportunism in evolution. *Am. Anthropol.* **81**, 818–840.

Niemeyer, C. L. and Anderson, J. R. (1983). Primate harassment of matings. *Ethol. Sociobiol.* **4**, 205–220.

Niemeyer, C. L. and Chamove, A. S. (1983). Motivation of harassment of matings in stump-tailed macaques. *Behaviour* **87**, 298–323.

Petit, O., Desportes, C. and Thierry, B. (1992). Differential probability of 'coproduction' in two species of macaque (*Macaca tonkeana, M. mulatta*). *Ethology* **90**, 107–120.

Pigliucci, M. and Kaplan, J. (2000). The fall and rise of Dr Pangloss: Adaptationism and the *Spandrels* paper 20 years later. *Trends Ecol. Evol.* **15**, 66–70.

Putnam, H. (1981). *Reason, Truth and Reality*. Cambridge: Cambridge University Press.

Quiatt, D. (1979). Aunts and mothers: adaptive implications of allomaternal behavior of nonhuman primates. *Am. Anthropol.* **81**, 310–319.

Rowell, T. E. (1979). How would we know if social organization were *not* adaptive? In *Primate Ecology and Human Origins*, ed. I. S. Bernstein and E. O. Smith. New York: Garland Press, pp. 1–22.

Sade, D. S. (1972). A longitudinal study of social behavior in rhesus monkeys. In *The Functional and Evolutionary Biology of Primates*, ed. R. H. Tuttle. Chicago, IL: Aldine Press, pp. 378–398.

Schubert, G. (1982). Infanticide by usurper Hanuman langur monkeys: a sociobiological myth. *Soc. Sci. Information* **21**, 199–244.

Sherman, P. J. (1988). The levels of analysis. *Anim. Behav.* **36**, 616–619.

Sommer, V. (2000). The holy wars about infanticide: which side are you on? and why? In *Infanticide by Males and its Implications*, ed. C. P. van Schaik and C. H. Janson. Cambridge: Cambridge University Press, pp. 9–26.

Stanford, C. B. (1992). Costs and benefits of allomothering in wild capped langurs (*Presbytis pileata*). *Behav. Ecol. Sociobiol.* **30**, 29–34.

Strier, K. B. (2000). *Primate Behavioral Ecology*. Needham Heights, MA: Allyn & Bacon.

Thierry, B. (1986a). Affiliative interference in mounts in a group of Tonkean macaques (*Macaca tonkeana*). *Am. J. Primatol.* **11**, 89–97.

(1986b). A comparative study of aggression and response to aggression in three species of macaque. In *Primate Ontogeny, Cognition, and Social Behaviour*, ed. J. G. Else and P. C. Lee. Cambridge: Cambridge University Press, pp. 307–313.

(1994). Emergence of social organisations in non-human primates. *Rev. Int. Systémique* **8**, 65–77.

(1997). Adaptation and self-organisation in primate societies. *Diogenes* **180**, 39–71.

(2000). Covariation of conflict management patterns across macaque species. In *Natural Conflict Resolution*, ed. F. Aureli and F. B. M. de Waal. Berkeley, CA: University of California Press, pp. 106–128.

Thierry, B., Gauthier, C. and Peignot, P. (1990). Social grooming in Tonkean macaques (*Macaca tonkeana*). *Int. J. Primatol.* **11**, 357–375.

Thierry, B., Anderson, J. R., Demaria, C. Desportes, C. and Petit, O. (1994). Tonkean macaque behaviour from the perspective of the evolution of Sulawesi macaques. In *Current Primatology*, vol. 2, ed. J. J. Roeder, B. Thierry, J. R. Anderson and N. Herrenschmidt. Strasbourg: Université Louis Pasteur, pp. 103–117.

Tutin, C. E. G. (1979). Responses of chimpanzees to copulation, with special reference to interference by immature individuals. *Anim. Behav.* **27**, 845–854.

van Schaik, C. P. (2000). Infanticide by male primates: the sexual selection hypothesis revisited. In *Infanticide by Males and its Implications*, ed. C. P. van Schaik and C. H. Janson. Cambridge: Cambridge University Press, pp. 27–60.

Williams, G. C. (1966). *Adaptation and Natural Selection*. Princeton, NJ: Princeton University Press.

7

Self-organisation in language

BART DE BOER
Vrije Universiteit Brussel

Definition of self-organisation

Many papers that describe processes resembling self-organisation according to the definition used here do not explicitly use the term 'self-organisation'. Instead terms like 'emergent behaviour', 'population dynamics', 'bifurcations', 'catastrophes' and others are used. In this chapter, such work will be subsumed under self-organisation. There might be slight differences in the phenomena that are described, but the basic ideas are the same, and an overview of this kind of work would be incomplete if attention was focused on only those papers that contain the term self-organisation.

Another reason why the term self-organisation is not used more frequently might be that the term itself is ill-defined. Different authors use different interpretations of the term. A selection of linguistic papers with self-organisation in the title (Lindblom *et al.*, 1984; Wildgen, 1990; Steels, 1995; Ehala, 1996; Demolin and Soquet, 1999; de Boer, 2000; Nicolis *et al.*, 2000) all have a slightly different view on what it is and what role it plays. Further, the term self-organisation might not be popular among linguists, because it has the negative connotation of being vague.

It is therefore useful and instructive to study in some more depth the definition of self-organisation used here. Self-organisation, according to this definition is 'The emergence of order on a global scale through interactions on a local scale.' The definition assumes there is a system that has two main components:

Self-Organisation and Evolution of Social Systems, ed. Charlotte K. Hemelrijk.
Published by Cambridge University Press. © Cambridge University Press 2005.

actors[1] and interactions. There is a population of actors, and the interactions always entail a number of actors that is considerably smaller than the total number of actors in the population. This is what is meant by interaction on a local scale. It has been mentioned above that the local and global scales, as well as the nature of the actors and interactions as well as their timescales can be interpreted in many different ways. The definition is therefore applicable to many aspects of language.

There are a number of notions that are sometimes used in conjunction with self-organising systems. These terms include the notions of chaos, bifurcations, emergence, attractors, catastrophes and (positive) feedback. A number of these terms have strict mathematical definitions and should therefore be used with care; as it is unlikely that all the conditions of the mathematical definition are fulfilled, such terms can only be used metaphorically in the context of language. This is not necessarily a bad thing, but one should not confuse the use of such terms with mathematical rigour.

Attractors, chaos, bifurcations and possibly catastrophes are rigorously defined mathematical terms that can only be used metaphorically when talking about language. In the context of language, attractors can be interpreted as stable states towards which languages tend to evolve. Language universals are sometimes considered to be attractors. Bifurcations and catastrophes can be used to describe linguistic events in which the organisation of a language – either in an individual or a population and either of a language's sound system, lexicon, grammar or another aspect – changes relatively suddenly. Chaos is often used to describe any unpredictable behaviour, and although it is true that languages, and social systems in general, sometimes show sensitivity to initial conditions, one should be very careful in using the term chaos, as unpredictable behaviour can have other causes as well, such as complex input from outside, real randomness or complex acyclic behaviour.

The notions of emergence and positive feedback are more useful in the description of language. Emergence and emergent behaviour are generally used to describe behaviour that cannot be predicted directly from the behaviours of individual actors in a system, but that is caused by interaction between actors and/or their environment. When emergent behaviour involves many individuals and results in regular collective behaviour, the behaviour is said to be self-organising. In order for this to happen there must be positive feedback between the behaviour of individuals. Small fluctuations in individuals must be amplified

---

[1] The use of the term 'actors' does not imply that these can necessarily determine their own actions. Actors can be neurons or even individual molecules, which behave in a completely reactive fashion.

and adopted by other individuals for a pattern to spread through the population. Self-amplifying behaviour is said to show positive feedback.

In language, emergence and positive feedback can be illustrated by the emergence of new words for new objects. At first, many words will be coined, but the ones that are most frequently used (or most frequently used by the most prestigious speakers) will be most useful in communication and will eventually be adopted by more and more speakers, until only one word remains.

History of self-organisation in language research

Probably the first time self-organisation was mentioned in the title of a linguistic publication was in the 1984 paper 'Self-organising processes and the explanation of language universals', by Lindblom, MacNeilage and Studdert-Kennedy (Lindblom *et al.*, 1984). Also in the early 1980s, ideas very close to self-organisation were being investigated in the field of dynamic linguistics (e.g. Altmann, 1985; Ballmer, 1985 and references therein) and catastrophe theory (Petitot-Cocorda, 1985). However, the ideas on which such work is based can be traced as far back as Zipf (1935). Zipf was possibly the first to propose within modern linguistics that linguistic structures emerge from the dynamics of language use. Of course, the term self-organisation had not been invented at that time, and so was not applied to this process.

Recently, emergent phenomena and self-organisation in language have received more attention, because user-friendly computing power has become available to language researchers. This makes it possible to test the consequences of complex theories about language in a population. Lindblom *et al.*'s (1984) paper describes computer modelling of a system of syllables, and is probably the first paper to link self-organisation in language and computer modelling. Liljencrants and Lindblom's (1972) paper had already followed a very similar methodology, but it did not talk about self-organisation. However, these models consider self-organisation within the sound system of a language, not in a population of language-users. The first computer models to use populations of language-users are by Hurford (1987, 1989) but these models consider the emergence of linguistic properties more as a result of evolution than of self-organisation. Other early work on population models of emergence of communication was reported by MacLennan (1992) and Werner and Dyer (1992) but these models focused on emergence of communication systems rather than language. Starting approximately in the mid-1990s, the number of articles on computer modelling of self-organising language systems increased rapidly (Batali, 1994; Kirby, 1994; Hashimoto and Ikegami, 1995; Steels, 1995; de Boer, 1997). Since then a number of collections of articles have appeared, mostly in the context of evolution of language, e.g. Hurford *et al.* (1998), Knight *et al.* (2000) and Cangelosi and Parisi (2002).

An example of self-organisation in language

It is well known that when languages use a certain place of articulation in their sound system (for example the alveolar ridge, used to produce sounds such as /t/, /d/, /n/ etc.), stop consonants tend to occur in both voiced and unvoiced versions. Thus, if a language uses /t/, it is very likely also to use /d/. If it has /p/ it will usually also have /b/, etc. This is not universally so, however. There are languages that do not use the distinction between voiced and unvoiced stop consonants, such as many Australian aboriginal languages, for example Yidiny (Dixon, 1977) or Dyirbal (Dixon, 1972). But such languages are rare.

This phenomenon can be explained using the view of language as a self-organising system in a population of language users. Whenever a language loses the distinction between voiced and unvoiced stop consonants, (such as the distinction between /t/ and /d/) there will be no more words that can be changed in meaning by changing a /t/ into a /d/ or vice versa. Then language-users are in principle free to use these sounds in free variation (although this might not occur, because doing so might be considered incorrect speech behaviour). When such free variation occurs, it is more likely that a stop consonant that is sandwiched between two vowels becomes voiced (thus the pronunciation /ada/ will be preferred over the pronunciation /ata/), while a stop consonant at the beginning or end of a word will become unvoiced (thus the pronunciation /ta/ will be preferred over /da/). This is just the consequence of what is easier to pronounce in rapid, casual speech.

Now, children learning the language will be exposed to these easy-to-pronounce variants more often, and will come to prefer them in their own speech production. Thus, in actual use, the language will have words with /d/, such as /ada/ and words with /t/, such as /ta/. Still, /d/ and /t/ cannot make a difference in meaning, as there are no words whose meaning changes by only changing a /d/ into a /t/. The use of either /d/ or /t/ can be predicted from the context.

But when the language changes, and through phonetic erosion loses the first syllable of bisyllabic words, words like /ada/ will turn into /da/. However, the language still has the word /ta/, and therefore a minimal pair is created, and the language will again have both /t/ and /d/ as speech sounds. As this process is much more rapid and likely than the process of losing the distinction between voiced and unvoiced sounds, the majority of the world's languages uses both voiced and unvoiced sounds.

This is an example of a linguistic explanation that uses actions of and inter-actions between individuals to explain the structure of language as a whole and is therefore an example of self-organisation in language.

Self-organisation on different levels

As mentioned above, self-organisation in language can occur in many different forms. It can occur in the organisation of language in the brain or in a population of language-users. It can be invoked to explain language universals, but also to explain how language changes and how language originated. Finally, self-organisation can occur in all aspects of language, from its sound system to meanings of words.

Self-organisation in a language-user's brain

Self-organisation in the brain is probably best known from the emergence of ocular dominance columns (see e.g. Erwin *et al.*, 1995). However, it is possible that it plays a role in the way language is organised in the brain as well. Lindblom *et al.* (1984) have proposed that self-organisation causes speech sounds to be organised in a phonemic (combinatorial) way instead of in a holistic way. They optimised systems of consonant–vowel syllables for acoustic distinctiveness and articulatory ease and found that this caused a limited number (of the available possible ones) of consonants and vowels to be used in a combinatorial way. They also found co-articulatory effects that resembled those that are found in human languages.

It seems that this work has remained relatively isolated. However, recently work on computer simulations has been published (Oudeyer, 2001) that investigates emergent structure and self-organisation in systems of speech sounds with a focus on what happens in an individual language-user. But this work takes interactions between language-users into account as well. The main problem with modelling self-organisation of language in the brain is that extremely little is known about how language is learned and stored on the neural level.

Self-organisation in a population of language-users

Most of the recent work on self-organisation and emergent phenomena in language has focused on populations of language-users. Such work has been on almost all aspects of language, including sound systems, grammar, lexicon formation, semantics and language change. A lot of this work focuses on evolution of language, but such work has relevance to the study of the role of self-organisation in language as well.

The basic idea behind this kind of work is that properties of language can be explained as a result of interactions between the individual language-users in addition to the properties and capacities of each individual language-user. In this respect this approach differs substantially from the approach to the study of language as proposed by De Saussure (1987) and later Chomsky (1965) where language is seen as abstract knowledge of an individual. The form in which language actually appears (called 'parole' by De Saussure and 'performance' by Chomsky) is seen as secondary. In the study of language as a self-organising system in a population, the use and appearance of language in daily use is seen as equally important to understanding what language is and what form it can take as the linguistic representations in the brain (see e.g. Steels, 1998a). Also, the distinction between diachronic linguistics (the study of how language changes) and synchronic linguistics (the study of the grammar of an individual language as well as the study of the human capacities for language) becomes less meaningful. Traditionally, these two branches have been separate and from the point of view of certain formal theories language change was even seen as problematic. However, when one views language as a self-organising system in a population, it becomes clear that one cannot study the one without the other. Of course, most linguists have realised this as well, but because of the complexity of the interactions and mechanisms involved it has not been possible to study it properly. More recently, linguistic work has started using elements of self-organisation and dynamics in the population (see e.g. Silverman, 2000).

Self-organisation of language in a population can be studied on many levels of detail. Some work focuses mainly on the interactions between transmission and learning of language (e.g. Kirby, 2001), some work uses larger populations of more realistic agents (e.g. Steels, 1998b) and even robots (Vogt, 2000). On the other hand, some work uses simpler mathematical models in order to understand the basic mechanisms (Nicolis et al., 2000). Other work takes the point of view that language in a population is subject to a kind of cultural evolution towards near-optimal solutions to the problem of communication under constraints (Redford et al., 2001).

What all these models have in common is that they view language (and therefore the universal properties of language) as the solution to the problem of communicating information and transferring the language from one generation to the next under constraints of speech production, perception and learning. They are therefore inherently dynamic: linguistic variations between individuals and populations as well as language change are considered to be inevitable outcomes. In this respect this view of language is more 'complete' than the view of language as knowledge of an individual.

Of course, taking the population dynamics into account in a theory of language makes it much more complicated and makes it a lot harder to make predictions on the basis of the theory and to test these predictions. For this reason, computer models are almost universally used to investigate these models.

Self-organisation and diachronic/synchronic linguistics

Systems of self-organisation in language are inherently a synthesis of synchronic and diachronic views of language. Some research, however, has focused more on one aspect than on the other.

Diachronic work

As models of self-organisation in language are inherently dynamic, they are not only very well suited to investigating language change, but also to investigating the origins of language. Models of language as an emergent property of a population of agents that needs to communicate can be used to find answers to such questions as: under what conditions will language emerge? What form will such a language take? Will only one language emerge, or will linguistic diversity be an emergent property of the system? Most recent research that sees language as a self-organising system has looked at the origins of language (e.g. see contributions in Hurford et al., 1998; Knight et al., 2000).

There is a small body of work, however, that looks mostly at the explanation of language change and linguistic diversity (Ehala, 1996; Livingstone and Fyfe, 1999; Nettle, 1999). Such models investigate the questions of how language can change over time and how a homogeneous language can split into multiple distinct languages. Such questions cannot be answered, and might even appear problematic when only looking at language as the capacity of an individual. From the perspective of language as a self-organising system in a population, such questions can be investigated. Again, because of the complexity of the models, computer simulations are used.

Synchronic work

Most of the work that has looked at self-organisation in language has focused on grammar (e.g. Batali, 1994; Kirby, 1994; Hashimoto and Ikegami, 1995; Steels, 1998b). However, all aspects of language have been investigated. The earliest work mentioning self-organisation focused on sound systems (Lindblom et al., 1984) and more recently new work has appeared on this subject (Berrah et al., 1996; de Boer, 1997, 2000; Berrah and Laboissière, 1999; Demolin and Soquet, 1999; Nicolis et al., 2000; Oudeyer, 2001; Redford et al., 2001). Lexicon formation has received a lot of attention as well (e.g. Oliphant, 1996; Steels, 1995) while formation of concepts (meanings) has been a topic of investigation, too (e.g. Hurford, 1989; Steels, 1995; Vogt, 2000). Morphology has received rather little attention, but there are some papers discussing this topic (e.g. Batali, 1998; Kirby, 2001).

Most of this work focuses on the role of self-organisation in a population of language-users; how it causes language to become coherent, and how it causes language to show certain universal tendencies as the result of interactions between individual language-users under constraints of perception, production and learning. These aspects can be investigated for each aspect of language separately, and this causes models to remain relatively simple. However, more realistic models must clearly take into account the interactions between different aspects of language, such as the influence of articulatory simplification on erosion of morphology and thus syntax. So far, little work has taken this into account, although especially Steels's (e.g. 1998a, b) work stresses that the interactions between the different levels of language are extremely important.

Computer modelling of self-organisation in language

As has been stressed several times, computer modelling is crucial for investigating self-organisation in language. It is only because so much computing power has recently come to the desktop of the average researcher that research into self-organisation in language has taken off to such an extent. Nevertheless, existing computers are not sufficiently powerful to model all complexities of language. It is therefore crucial for successful computer simulations to use the right kinds of simplification. Finding such simplifications is the biggest challenge for designing a good computer simulation.

It is, however, impossible to give guidelines about which simplifications to make. It all depends on which aspect of language is to be investigated, and whether one wants to explain abstract properties of language (e.g. if compositionality is a necessary outcome of language evolution) or whether one wants to investigate a more specific question about language (e.g. why certain vowels occur more frequently than others or why more frequently occurring verbs tend to be irregular). In any case, simplifications must fulfil two criteria: they must not qualitatively change the problem under investigation and there must be a mapping from the simplified system to real language. Qualitative changes could occur, for example, if the computational complexity of a learning model is exponential in the length of utterances, or if the simulation depends on agents transferring or sharing information in an unspecified (telepathic) way.

Computer models of populations of language-users can be constructed in different ways. It is possible to make extremely simplified, almost mathematical models in order to study general behaviour of language in a population. In such models, there is no need to model a real population, but only certain variables that describe general properties (such as the fraction of agents that have a certain linguistic trait) of the language. These models are simple to build and investigate, and it is often possible to prove mathematical properties of their behaviour. However, such models can of necessity provide only a limited insight in the dynamics of self-organisation in language.

More sophisticated models model a real population of 'agents' (abstract models of language-users) that each have the ability to produce, perceive and learn certain aspects (i.e. sounds, words, grammatical rules, etc.) of language. The way in which these agents operate and learn does not necessarily have to be modelled directly on the way the human brain works. Some models are based on neural network implementations (e.g. Batali, 1998) but most of the work cited here uses higher-level, symbolic approaches. This is all right, as the focus of this work is to investigate the dynamics of language in a population. One should just be careful not to equip the agents with capabilities that are biologically impossible.

Interactions between agents are implemented directly, and the system is iterated through a large number of interactions. Often this approach allows for a dynamic population: agents can be inserted into and removed from the population in order to implement realistic population dynamics. Also, spatial structure can be given to the population: agents have a spatial location, and agents that are closer together have a higher probability of interacting than agents further apart. Furthermore, the world in which the agents operate and about which they communicate can be made more complicated. Many models have only a fixed number of meanings, or only abstract meanings about which the agents can communicate, but other models have the agents communicate about a more elaborately modelled world, or even about the real world as observed through video cameras (Steels, 1998b).

Another way of implementing populations in a computer model is in the form of a genetic algorithm (Batali, 1994; Hashimoto and Ikegami, 1995; Zuidema and Hogeweg, 2000). Such a model works like biological evolution in nature. Individuals get assigned a fitness on the basis of their behaviour, and their likelihood of creating offspring is proportional to their fitness. Offspring will be like their parents, but there is a possibility of mutation and random recombination of genetic information from the parents. Fitness in linguistic models can for example be evaluated by the ability of the individuals to parse sentences, to produce or perceive sounds or to communicate about the environment. Although self-organisation can occur in such models, and although such work is closely related to research into emergent behaviour and self-organisation, in general there is an element of global control in such evolutionary models. Unless the function by which individuals are evaluated also evolves (this would be co-evolution) it has a global influence that falls outside the definition of a self-organising system. However, the results of these simulations do have relevance for the study of language as a self-organising system, and so they cannot be excluded in this discussion.

The most sophisticated models combine evolution and self-organisation in a population. The individuals are evaluated by how well they learn the language, but as the language changes because of self-organisation in the population, the evaluation function is no longer static, but changes with the changing system. However, such systems would be computationally extremely complex, and it appears that so far only plans exist to build such systems, but none has been realised.

An example of self-organisation

The example that will be presented here is from my own work on self-organisation in vowel systems, and has been published more completely in de Boer (1997, 2000, 2001). It fits in the tradition of investigating vowel systems with computer models (e.g. Liljencrants and Lindblom, 1972; Schwartz et al., 1997b) and is more directly based on two artificial life models of vowel system transfer (Berrah et al., 1996; Glotin and Laboissière, 1996). At its basis lies the observation that vowel systems in human languages show remarkable regularities (e.g. Crothers, 1978; Schwartz et al., 1997a).

Although humans can produce and distinguish many different vowel sounds, human languages tend to use only a limited subset of these. At least 45 different qualities are recognised by phoneticians (Ladefoged and Maddieson, 1996) and languages can make use of up to at least 15 of these at the same time (Maddieson, 1984; Schwartz et al., 1997a). Some languages are said to have more vowels, but they make use of secondary distinctions, such as vowel length, nasalisation, etc. However, in the large majority of human languages, vowel systems tend to be quite small and tend to be constructed among relatively simple rules. The most frequently occurring number of vowels in human languages is five, and these vowels are almost always /i/, /e/, /a/, /o/ and /u/. An example of a language with such a vowel system is Spanish. Moreover, most of the world's languages contain the vowels /i/, /a/ and /u/, and there is a small repertoire of (about eight to ten) vowels that accounts for most of the vowel sounds occurring in the world's languages. Only when vowel repertoires become really large are more exotic speech sounds used, such as the rounded front vowels /y/, /ø/ and /œ/ that are found in French, German and the Scandinavian languages. Coincidentally,

Western and Northern Europe are areas where languages with extraordinarily many vowel sounds are spoken, and English is one of these. In this respect English is quite unusual.

But there is yet another remarkable property of human vowel systems. They tend to be symmetrical. If a language contains, for example, the vowel /o/ it is more likely than expected on the ground of the a priori probability, also to contain the vowel /e/. This vowel corresponds in tongue height, but is articulated in the front part of the mouth, instead of in the back. Similar symmetries are found for many different pairs of vowels.

Traditionally (Jakobson and Halle, 1956), and within the tradition of generative grammar (Chomsky and Halle, 1968), these regularities have been explained as the result of innate properties of the human brain, and more specifically the human language faculty. But one can ask whether it is really necessary to postulate innate feature detectors and preferences to explain the regularities. Liljencrants and Lindblom (1972) have shown that one would expect to find such regularities in systems that are optimised for acoustic distance between the individual vowels. They built a computer simulation that optimised the distance between a given number of points representing vowels in an acoustic space. From this computer simulation emerged vowel systems that resembled the most frequent systems found in human languages. Subsequent refinements of this model (e.g. Schwartz *et al.*, 1997b) have shown even better correspondence with human language data.

The question remains, however, how vowel systems become optimised. No individual language-learner optimises. In fact, infants are very good at learning the subtlest distinctions in vowel quality. Also, there are languages with vowel systems that are far from optimal, but these are learned perfectly well. Apparently the cause of optimisation is not to be found in the individual infant's learning behaviour.

Within the framework of self-organisation, an alternative hypothesis can be formulated. Perhaps the optimisation is the result of repeated interactions between agents that learn and use vowels under constraints of speech production, perception and learning? This hypothesis has been investigated using a computer model (de Boer, 1997, 2000, 2001). This computer model can only be described very briefly here; for details the reader is referred to the original references.

The model is based on a population of agents that can each produce, perceive and learn vowels in a realistic way. Each agent has a simple speech synthesiser that can generate all basic vowels, based on three inputs: the tongue height, tongue position and lip rounding needed to articulate the vowel. Thus for an /i/, the tongue needs to be high and to the front and the lips need to be spread, while for an /o/, the tongue needs to be somewhere between high and low, but to the back of the mouth, and the lips need to be rounded. These three parameters are sufficient for generating all basic vowel qualities. Vowels are stored as 'prototypes'. For each vowel an agent knows, a point in both acoustic and articulatory space is stored that is most representative of that particular vowel. Perception is based on a cognitively plausible distance function that is based on properties of the sound spectrum of the vowels. For a given signal, its distance is calculated to all acoustic prototypes, and the one with the shortest distance is defined to be the vowel recognised. Agents start out with empty vowel repertoires, and add and remove vowels on the basis of the interactions with other agents. In order to get the games started, and in order to put pressure on the agents to extend their repertoires, agents can add random new vowels with low probability (1% per game).

The agents interact in so-called imitation games. In each imitation game, two agents are chosen randomly from the population. One agent chooses a random vowel from its repertoire and produces this, while adding noise. The other agent analyses this sound in terms of its prototypes, and picks the one that is closest to the signal. It then produces the corresponding sound in turn, also adding noise. The first agent then analyses this sound in terms of its prototypes, and checks whether the prototype it recognises is the one it originally used for producing the sound. If this is the case, the game is said to be successful. If not, it is a failure. This is communicated to the other agents through 'non-verbal feedback'. Of course, in reality children do not get feedback (non-verbal or other) about the sounds they produce. However, one could imagine that infants derive information from things such as emotional state of the interlocutor or failure to achieve a certain communicative goal.

As a reaction on the imitation game, agents update their vowel system. They can add a vowel if necessary – this happens especially often in the beginning of the game when agents' repertoires are empty and new vowels are added as close approximations of heard signals. Also, agents sometimes add random vowels, in order to create pressure to increase the size of their repertoires or to get imitation started when an agent's repertoire is empty and it has to produce a sound nevertheless. Vowels can also be discarded if it turns out that they are not successful for imitating other agents' vowels. This is evaluated on the basis of their past success or failure in imitation games. Vowels can also be merged if they come too close together in either acoustic or articulatory space. Finally, agents can shift vowels in their repertoire over a small distance in order to approximate more closely the signal heard in the imitation game. These updates to an agent's vowel repertoire are not directly inspired by the way children learn. However, they are biologically plausible in principle, as they only involve

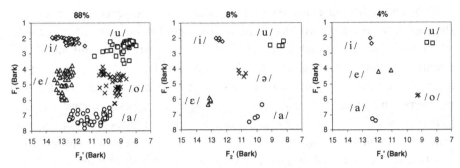

Figure 7.1 Emergent five-vowel systems, classified for configuration type. The acoustic space is based on the frequencies of the first two main peaks in the vowel's frequency spectrum (called F_1 and F_2') and these are plotted in the logarithmic 'Bark' frequency scale. Distance in the Bark frequency scale corresponds better to perceptual distance than in the Hertz frequency scale. The plots are structured in such a way that vowels appear in positions in which phoneticians usually plot them: high front vowels to the upper left, low back vowels to the lower right.

simple manipulations and local information. Human infants probably use more powerful statistical learning techniques, but for simplicity's sake, a learning model that was as simple and transparent as possible was used.

All these actions and interactions lead to the emergence of realistic vowel systems. It turns out that these vowel systems are not only remarkably like the vowel systems found in human languages, but that the frequency with which different types of vowel systems occur agrees remarkably well with the frequency in which they occur in human languages. An example of this is given in Fig. 7.1. In this figure, five-vowel systems that emerged are classified according to the configuration of vowels in the systems. In 49 out of 100 populations that had the same parameter settings, five-vowel systems emerged (four- and six-vowel systems also emerged). Systems with similar configurations (determined on the basis of the number of front, back and central vowels, as well as their symmetry) are grouped together in the same figure. Each vowel system emerged in a population of 20 agents. From each of the populations, one agent was selected randomly, and this agent was used to represent that population's vowel system. The vowel systems of all agents with the same configuration were plotted together in acoustic space. Thus, each data point per cluster belongs to a different agent in a different population, while for every agent five data points (each indicated with a different symbol) appear in the figure.

It can be observed that the frequencies of the emerged vowel systems correspond quite well with those found in human languages. In Schwartz *et al.*'s (1997a) survey, 89% of the vowel systems were like the ones in the leftmost frame, and both other types of system occurred in 5% of the languages in their sample.

As has been defined above, self-organisation is the emergence of global order through local interactions. The local interactions in this simulation consist of imitation games. In each game only two agents participate, and only local updates are made to an agent's vowel system (no global optimisation is performed). The emerging global order consists of concentrated clusters of vowel prototypes that are shared in a population of agents. The possible vowel systems that emerge are restricted to a reasonably small class of realistic vowel systems. Note that the emerged vowel systems are not necessarily completely optimal. The fact that the agents need to have a vowel system that is similar to the systems used by the other agents in the population may cause the system to stay stuck in a local optimum. This is reminiscent of the situation in human languages, where suboptimal vowel systems also occur from time to time. Here too, a vowel system can become suboptimal due to the history of the language. However, single language users cannot change the system too much towards optimality, as this would make him or her incomprehensible for the other speakers. On the basis of these and similar results, it can be concluded that self-organisation in a population under constraints of perception, production and learning can explain the universal tendencies of human vowel systems; no specific innate tendencies are necessary.

Conclusion

This chapter has presented an overview of work on language as a self-organising system. It has been shown that viewing language in this way is extremely useful. Self-organisation is the emergence of global order through interactions on a local scale. It can happen (and has been investigated) in the human brain, but most work into self-organisation in language has focused on linguistic phenomena in a population of language-users.

Self-organisation provides a means by which diachronic linguistics (the description of how language changes) can be unified with synchronic linguistics (the description of grammars of human languages and the capacities that humans bring to bear on the tasks of learning and understanding language). Self-organisation can be used to gain insight in such diverse aspects of language as phonological universals of sound systems, the emergence of grammar, linguistic change or the way a population of language-users adopts new words. All these approaches have in common that they view language as a dynamic system in which interactions between language-users is as important as the knowledge and capacities of those language-users. In this respect models of self-organisation attach equal importance to both De Saussure's 'langue' and 'parole', and Chomsky's 'performance' and 'competence'.

As theories of self-organisation in language involve extremely complex dynamics, most of the work uses computer simulations. However, this reliance on the computer makes it more difficult for traditional linguists to understand and contribute to this work. Perhaps because of this, a lot of work on language and self-organisation has been published in non-linguistic journals and conference proceedings.

Much work has already been done on language as a self-organising system, and this area of study is rapidly expanding. However, many extremely interesting experiments still remains to be done. An important task for researchers of self-organisation in language remains to make their work accessible to the large community of linguists that are less literate in computers.

Acknowledgement

This article was written at the AI-lab of the Vrije Universiteit, Brussels. The author wishes to thank Willem Zuidema for suggestions about literature.

References

Altmann, G. (1985). On the dynamic approach to language. In *Linguistic Dynamics*, ed. T. T. Ballmer. Berlin, Walter de Gruyter, pp. 181–189.

Ballmer, T. T. (1985). *Linguistic Dynamics*. Berlin: Walter de Gruyter.

Batali, J. (1994). Innate biases and critical periods: combining evolution and learning in the acquisition of syntax. In *Proc. 4th Artificial Life Workshop*, ed. R. Brooks and P. Maes. Cambridge, MA: MIT Press, pp. 160–171.

(1998). Computational simulations of the emergence of grammar. In *Approaches to the Evolution of Language*, ed. J. R. Hurford, M. Studdert-Kennedy and C. Knight. Cambridge: Cambridge University Press, pp. 405–426.

Berrah, A.-R. and Laboissière, R. (1999). SPECIES: an evolutionary model for the emergence of phonetic structures in an artificial society of speech agents. In *Advances in Artificial Life, Lecture Notes in Artificial Intelligence*, ed. D. Floreano, J.-D. Nicoud and F. Mondada. Berlin: Springer-Verlag, pp. 674–678.

Berrah, A.-R., Glotin, H., Laboissière, R., Bessière, P. and Boë, L.-J. (1996). From form to formation of phonetic structures: an evolutionary computing perspective. In *Proc. ICML 1996 Workshop on Evolutionary Computing and Machine Learning*, Bari, Italy, pp. 23–29.

Cangelosi, A. and Parisi, D. (2002). *Simulating the Evolution of Language*. London: Springer-Verlag.

Chomsky, N. (1965). *Aspects of the Theory of Syntax*. Cambridge, MA: MIT Press.

Chomsky, N. and Halle, M. (1968). *The Sound Pattern of English*. Cambridge, MA: MIT Press.

Crothers, J. (1978). Typology and universals of vowel systems. In *Universals of Human Language*, vol. 2, *Phonology*, ed. J. H. Greenberg, C. A. Ferguson and E. A. Moravcsik. Stanford, CA: Stanford University Press, pp. 93–152.

de Boer, B. (1997). Generating vowels in a population of agents. In *Proc. 4th European Conf. Artificial Life*, ed. P. Husbands and I. Harvey. Cambridge, MA: MIT Press, pp. 503–510.

(2000). Self-organisation in vowel systems. *J. Phonet.* **28**, 441–465.

(2001). *The Origins of Vowel Systems.* Oxford: Oxford University Press.

Demolin, D. and Soquet, A. (1999). The role of self-organisation in the emergence of phonological systems. *Evol. Communication* 3, 21–48.

De Saussure, F. (1987). (ed. T. de Mauro). *Cours de Linguistique Générale.* Paris: Payot.

Dixon, R. M. W. (1972). *The Dyirbal Language of North Queensland.* Cambridge: Cambridge University Press.

(1977). *A Grammar of Yidiny.* Cambridge: Cambridge University Press.

Ehala, M. (1996). Self-organisation and language change. *Diachronica* 13, 1–28.

Erwin, E., Obermayer, K. and Schulten, K. (1995). Models of orientation and ocular dominance columns in the visual cortex: a critical comparison. *Neur. Comput.* **7**, 425–468.

Glotin, H. and Laboissière, R. (1996). Emergence du code phonétique dans une société de robots parlants. *Actes de la Conférence de Rochebrune 1996: Du Collectif au social.* Paris: Ecole Nationale Supérieure des Télécommunications.

Hashimoto, T. and Ikegami, T. (1995). Evolution of symbolic grammar systems. In *Advances in Artificial Life, Lecture Notes in Artificial Intelligence*, ed. F. Morán, A. Moreno, J. J. Merelo and P. Chacón. Berlin: Springer-Verlag, pp. 812–823.

Hurford, J. R. (1987). *Language and Number.* Oxford: Blackwell Scientific Publications.

(1989). Biological evolution of the Sausurean sigan as a component of the language acquisition device, *Lingua* **77**, pp. 187–222.

Hurford, J. R., Studdert-Kennedy, M. and Knight, C. (1998). *Approaches to the Evolution of Language.* Cambridge: Cambridge University Press.

Jakobson, R. and Halle, M. (1956). *Fundamentals of Language.* The Hague: Mouton.

Kirby, S. (1994). Adaptive explanations for language universals: a model of Hawkins' performance theory. *Sprachtypol. Universalienforsch.* 47, 186–210.

(2001). Spontaneous evolution of linguistic structure: an iterated learning model of the emergence of regularity and irregularity. *IEEE Trans. Evol. Comput.* **5**, 102–110.

Knight, C., Studdert-Kennedy, M. and Hurford, J. R. (2000). *The Evolutionary Emergence of Language.* Cambridge: Cambridge University Press.

Ladefoged, P. and Maddieson, I. (1996). *The Sounds of the World's Languages.* Oxford: Blackwell Scientific Publications.

Liljencrants, L. and Lindblom, B. (1972). Numerical simulations of vowel quality systems: the role of perceptual contrast. *Language* **48**, 839–862.

Lindblom, B., MacNeilage, P. and Studdert-Kennedy, M. (1984). Self-organising processes and the explanation of language universals. In *Explanations for Language Universals*, ed. B. Butterworth, B. Comrie, and Ö. Dahl. Berlin: Walter de Gruyter, pp. 181–203.

Livingstone, D. and Fyfe, C. (1999). Modelling the evolution of linguistic diversity. In *Advances in Artificial Life, Lecture Notes in Artificial Intelligence*, ed. D. Floreano, J.-D. Nicoud and F. Mondada. Berlin: Springer-Verlag, pp. 704–708.

MacLennan, B. (1992). Synthetic ecology: an approach to the study of communication. In *Artificial Life*, vol. 2, ed. C. G. Langton, C. Taylor, J. D. Farmer and S. Rasmussen. Redwood City, CA: Addison-Wesley, pp. 631–658.

Maddieson, I. (1984). *Patterns of Sounds*. Cambridge: Cambridge University Press.

Nettle, D. (1999). *Linguistic Diversity*. Oxford: Oxford University Press.

Nicolis, S. C., Deneubourg, J. L., Soquet, A. and Demolin, D. (2000). Fluctuation induced self-organization of a phonological system. *Proceedings of International Conference on Complex Systems*, Nashua.

Oliphant, M. (1996) The dilemma of Saussurean communication. *Biosystems* 37, 31–38.

Oudeyer, P.-Y. (2001). Coupled neural maps for the origins of vowel systems. In *Proc. Int. Conf. Artificial Neural Networks 2001, Lecture Notes in Computer Science*, ed. G. Dorffner, H. Bischof, and K. Hornol. Berlin: Springer-Verlag, pp. 1171–1176.

Petitot-Cocorda, J. (1985). *Les catastrophes de la parole*. Paris: Maloine.

Redford, M. A., Chen, C. C. and Miikulainen, R. (2001). Constrained emergence of universals and variation in syllable systems. *Language and Speech* **44**, 27–56.

Schwartz, J. L., Boë, L. J., Vallée, N. and Abry, C. (1997a). Major trends in vowel system inventories. *J. Phonet.* **25**, 233–253.

(1997b). The dispersion–focalization theory of vowel systems. *J. Phonet.* **25**, 255–286.

Silverman, D. (2000). Hypotheses concerning the phonetic and functional origins of tone displacement in Zulu. *Stud. Afr. Linguist.* **29**, 1–32.

Steels, L. (1995). A self-organizing spatial vocabulary. *Artif. Life* **2**, 319–332.

(1998a). Synthesising the origins of language and meaning using co-evolution, self-organisation and level formation. In *Approaches to the Evolution of Language*, ed. J. R. Hurford, M. Studdert-Kennedy and C. Knight. Cambridge: Cambridge University Press, pp. 384–404.

(1998b). The origins of syntax in visually grounded robotic agents. *Artif. Intell.* **103**, 1–24.

Vogt, P. (2000). Bootstrapping grounded symbols by minimal autonomous robots. *Evol. Commun.* **4**, 89–118.

Werner, G. M. and Dyer, M. G. (1992). Evolution of communication in artificial organisms. In *Artificial Life*, vol. 2, ed. C. G. Langton, C. Taylor, J. D. Farmer and S. Rasmussen. Redwood City, CA: Addison-Wesley, pp. 659–687.

Wildgen, W. (1990). Basic principles of self-organisation in language. In *Synergetics of Cognition*, ed. H. Haken and M. Stadler. Berlin: Springer-Verlag, pp. 415–426.

Zipf, G. K. (1935). *The Psychobiology of Language*. Cambridge, MA: MIT Press.

Zuidema, W. and Hogeweg, P. (2000). Selective advantages of syntactic language: a model study. In *Proc. 22nd Ann. Mtg. Cognitive Science Society*, pp. 577–582.

8

Dictatorship effect of majority rule in voting in hierarchical systems

SERGE GALAM

Centre de Recherche en Epistémologie Appliquée (CREA), Paris

Introduction

In recent years statistical physics (Pathria, 1972; Ma, 1976) has been applied to a large spectrum of fields outside the scope of non-living matter (Bunde *et al.*, 2002). While applications to social sciences are growing, they are still scarce (de Oliveira *et al.*, 2000). In this chapter we analyse a basic ingredient of social organisations: the legitimacy of top leadership with respect to the distribution of support for various political trends present at the bottom of the organisation.

In hierarchical democratic systems each level is chosen from the one just below using a local majority rule. In principle this is supposed to yield 100% power to the larger trend. In the case of two competing trends, it means receiving more than 50% of the overall global support. This democratic ideal can seldom be satisfied, because the trend leading the organisation has several advantages. We show that accounting for such an asymmetry between the ruling trend and the challenging one may turn a democratic system into a drastic dictatorship.

This paradox is a consequence of the underlying dynamics associated with multi-level elections. It appears to obey a threshold-like dynamics, which can lead to democratic self-elimination of the huge majority against a minority trend which is in power (Galam, 1986). Indeed, repeated elections can drive the threshold for attaining power to a significant asymmetric value. For instance, it can be down to 23% for the group already in power and up to 77% for its challenging competitor.

Self-Organisation and Evolution of Social Systems, ed. Charlotte K. Hemelrijk.
Published by Cambridge University Press. © Cambridge University Press 2005.

These effects are universal and operate in most organisations that have more than just one hierarchical level. They provide a new explanation for the common observation that it is difficult to overthrow a ruling group. Therefore, we will determine the democratic conditions under which a small minority remains in power. Moreover, the recent drastic increase of the failure to vote by people in Western countries is demonstrated also to contribute to this shift away from 50% of the threshold to power.

At this stage it is worth stating that we aim to emphasise the existence of a social phenomenon associated with voting by the majority rule rather than to explain all details of democratic elections. Moreover we are focusing on committees of a small size. Indeed a similar process has been shown to make reforms difficult (Galam, 2000). A diffusive version has also been studied. There, instead of voting for representatives, the same people move in a two-dimensional space and meet in small groups to discuss an issue with some probability. Then, depending on the local majority within each group, people change their mind accordingly. The model was also applied to explain the emergence of new species (Galam et al., 1998) and was also extended to explain phenomena of rumours (Galam, 2002).

The chapter is organised as follows. In the next section we present the voting model in the case of two competing political trends A and B within one unique hierarchical system. No strategy is included. The case of three-person cells is studied first. It yields a critical threshold to power at 50% of overall support within the whole organization. Only a few voting levels are required to have no people elected from the minority trend of the organization. Next we introduce the advantage of being already in power. A bias is given to the ruling trend in the absence of a majority for even cells with four persons. Accordingly, the 2A-2B tie in voting is considered as being in favour of the ruling party. Such a bias is found to shift the value of the critical threshold to power from 50% to 77% for the opposition. Cell size effects of the threshold value are subsequently analysed (pp. 145–146), and a visualization of a numerical simulation (Galam and Wonczak, 2000) is shown (pp. 146–147). We then discuss the extension of the model to three competing trends. It appears that this enhances dictatorship effects. To conclude, the results of the model are compared to the historical collapse of eastern European communist parties during the last century.

The voting model

We start from an organisation with a leading policy denoted by A and a challenging policy B. Organisation members either support A or B, in the respective proportions p_0 and $1 - p_0$. Each person has an opinion. The system may be a political party, a firm, a social institution, etc.

We start by constituting a bottom-level hierarchy called level 0 from small-size cells created by an aggregation of people from the organisation. The process is done randomly. Once formed, each one of these cells elects one representative, either an A or a B, using a local majority rule within the cell.

The elected people form the first hierarchical level of the hierarchy, level 1. The process is then repeated again and again, each time starting from people elected at one level to form new cells, which in turn elect new representatives to build up a higher level just above. At the top level is the president. A pyramid-like structure is obtained (Fig. 8.1).

Considering three persons per bottom cell is the simplest case. People are randomly selected from the whole population. It could correspond to location of homes or work places. Each cell then elects a representative using a local majority rule. Cells with either 3A or 2A elect an A. Otherwise B is elected. All elected people constitute the hierarchy level 1. All these elected people are then distributed randomly among new cells of three persons each. Afterwards they elect new representatives, still using local majority rules to build the hierarchy level 2. The same process of cell forming and voting is repeated again and again up to the top of the hierarchy with the president, as shown in Fig. 8.1 (Galam, 1999).

According to the present model of three persons per group the probability of having an A elected at level $(n + 1)$ above level n is

$$p_{n+1} = p_n^3 + 3p_n^2(1 - p_n), \tag{8.1}$$

where p_n is the proportion of elected persons A at level n. It is a binomial law which has three fixed points 0, 1 and $\frac{1}{2}$. The first one corresponds to no A elected, the second one implies that only A is elected. Both are stable fixed points. It means that in their vicinity, the election process drives the respective probability towards them.

In contrast the last one is unstable. For the A trend it determines the threshold to either full power (at 1) or to total disappearance (at 0). Starting from $p_0 < \frac{1}{2}$ leads to extinction while $p_0 > \frac{1}{2}$ results in full power for A. Repeated voting by the majority rule produces the self-elimination of any proportion of A as long as the overall support is less than 50%. However this democratic self-elimination requires a sufficient number of voting levels to be completed. For instance starting from $p_0 = 0.43$ only two levels lead to $p_1 = 0.40$ and $p_2 = 0.35$. In this case, although B has 57% support within the whole organisation, they win the presidency with a probability of 65%. Therefore the building of a hierarchical structure has weakened the overall democratic feature of voting using

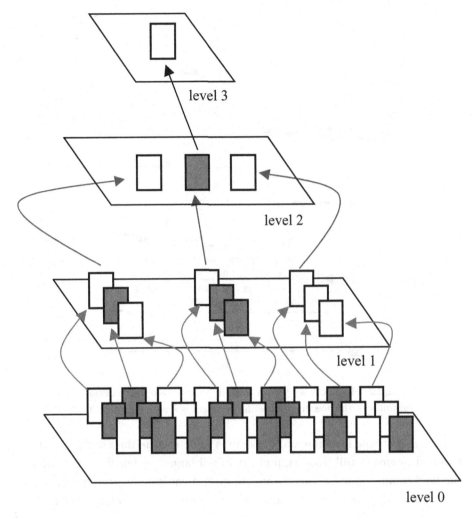

Figure 8.1 Illustration of a democratic hierarchy with three levels above the bottom one. Three persons form each cell. While people at the bottom are selected randomly from the whole organisation, people at higher levels have been elected. At the top (third level) is the president.

a majority rule since now the bottom majority is no longer sure of winning the presidency. This is shown in Fig. 8.2 truncated at only two levels above bottom.

To recover the democratic legitimacy of the system, more levels must be added as shown in Fig. 8.2. In this particular case, five additional levels are requested to ensure the presidency to the majority of the bottom level. Seven levels yield the series $p_0 = 0.43$, $p_1 = 0.40$, $p_2 = 0.35$, $p_3 = 0.28$, $p_4 = 0.20$, $p_5 = 0.10$, $p_6 = 0.03$, $p_7 = 0.00$.

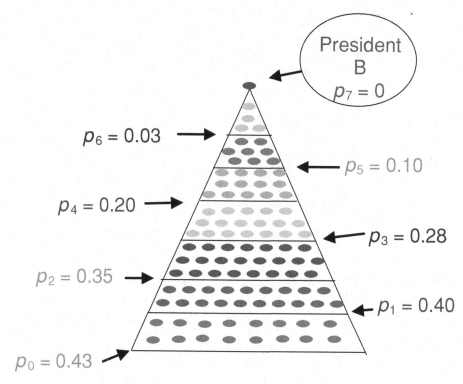

Figure 8.2 A hierarchy with seven levels in order to recover the democratic legitimacy of the presidency. Now the president is A with a probability of 100%.

At this stage the instrumental question is to determine the number of levels required to ensure full leadership to the initial larger tendency. To make sense the level number must be small enough, most organisations having only a few levels (fewer than 10). The calculation will be presented below (pp. 146–147).

Being in power

The advantage to be in power can be experienced in everyday life in any social organisation. The group holding the presidency has a definite advantage over any challenging group. The more local an election is, the stronger such an effect is. Various reasons can explain such an asymmetry. To try to single out the entire complex mechanisms involved in the phenomenon is rather difficult and clearly outside the scope of the present work. Instead, we can translate this asymmetry in a simple manner in our model. To account for an inertia to be in power we introduce the possibility of a tie in a voting cell by considering even groups of four persons each. In case of a tie at 2A–2B, an A representative is elected since trend A belongs to the current leading group.

Accordingly the probability at level n to get a B elected at level $n + 1$ is:

$$p_{n+1} = p_n^4 + 4p_n^3(1 - p_n),\qquad(8.2)$$

where p_n is as before the proportion of B persons elected at level n. In contrast for an A to be elected the probability is:

$$1 - p_{n+1} = (1 - p_n)^4 + 4(1 - p_n)^3 p_n + 2(1 - p)^2 p_n^2,\qquad(8.3)$$

where the last term embodies the bias in favour of A (a tie 2A–2B), the current ruling trend. From Eqs. (8.2) and (8.3) the stable fixed points are still 0 and 1. However the unstable one is now drastically shifted to $\frac{1+\sqrt{13}}{6} \approx 0.77$ for B (Eq. (8.2)) while it is ≈ 0.23 for A (Eq. (8.3)).

Running an election appears to be a drastically different challenge for the trend that wants to maintain power compared to the one that wants to take it over. Using an a priori reasonable bias in favour of A has altered the majority rule in democratic voting to lead to a dictatorship outcome. To get to power the A trend must pass over 77% of overall support which is almost out of reach in any normal situation.

In addition to the asymmetry the bias makes the number of levels before reaching democratic self-elimination even smaller than in the preceding case (three individuals per cell). Starting again from $p_0 = 0.45$ we now get $p_1 = 0.24$, $p_2 = 0.05$ and $p_3 = 0.00$. Instead of eight levels, now three are enough to make the B trend disappear from elected representatives. To illustrate the strength of the self-eliminating effect, let us start far above 50% with for instance $p_0 = 0.70$; the associated series then becomes $p_1 = 0.66$, $p_2 = 0.57$, $p_3 = 0.42$, $p_4 = 0.20$, $p_5 = 0.03$ and $p_6 = 0.00$. With only six levels of voting, 70% of support to a given challenging trend has shrunk to zero.

Size dependence effect

Up to now, we have considered very small groups per cell. But many organisations have larger groups per cell. Extending the model to any size r results in more complicated binomial equations. However the main features remain unchanged. For a cell of size r the function becomes

$$p_n = \sum_{l=r}^{m} \frac{r!}{l!(r-l)!} p_{n-1}^l (1 - p_{n-1})^{r-l}\qquad(8.4)$$

where $m = \frac{r+1}{2}$ for odd r and $m = \frac{r+2}{2}$ for even r ($m = 3$ at $r = 4$) which thus accounts for the bias in favour of the A trend.

From Eq. (8.4) it is found that the two stable fixed points 0 and 1 are unchanged. In the case of odd sizes, the unstable fixed point is also unchanged at $\frac{1}{2}$.

Table 8.1 *Cell size versus the*
threshold for taking over power for the
challenging trend

Cell size	Threshold
2	1
4	0.77
6	0.65
8	0.61
10	0.58
20	0.53
26	0.52

However, for even sizes, an asymmetry emerges between the threshold values for respectively rulers and their challengers. It is found to weaken with increasing sizes varying from $\frac{1+\sqrt{13}}{6} \approx 0.77$ at $r = 4$ towards $\frac{1}{2}$ but asymptotically from above. It remains significantly larger than $\frac{1}{2}$ for sizes larger than a dozen people as shown in Table 8.1.

In today's democratic countries differences between two competing trends are usually just a few percentage points. Therefore, even a small asymmetry as shown in Table 8.1 represents a very meaningful advantage for the ruling trend. Moreover it is worth noting that increasing cell size reduces the number of levels necessary to get to the stable fixed points making the dynamic of self-elimination faster.

The number of levels required to reach the presidency with certainty are not shown since they depend on the initial proportions of respective support at the bottom level.

Visualisation of a numerical simulation

To display the strength of the phenomena, we show two snapshots of a numerical simulation done on a square lattice with $64 \times 64 = 4096$ persons (Galam and Wonczak, 2000). The two tendencies, A and B, are represented respectively in white and black squares with the bias in favour of the black ones, i.e. a tied 2–2 vote becomes a black square. A structure with seven levels is shown. We can see on each picture how a huge majority of white squares eliminates itself.

Figure 8.3 shows a case with a huge 76.07% initial A (white) support. Now six levels are needed to get a black square (B) elected. The initial B support (black) to hold on power is at only 23.03%. In contrast, Fig. 8.4 shows a case with 77.05% initial A (white) support. Now the A trend (white) takes the presidency from the black trend.

Extension to three competing groups

Up to now we have treated the case of two competing trends. However, most real situations involve more than two competing groups. To study the robustness of our finding with respect to multi-trend competition, we consider the case of three competing groups, A, B and C, with cell size of three. This cell size was found to have a 50% threshold for two competing trends. No asymmetry was present.

However, while dealing with three distinct competing trends, there now exists a configuration with 1A–1B–1C, which yields no majority. Here the ruling trend cannot claim to take an advantage from such an undecided case. Instead the issue is usually set by bilateral agreement among the three trends, A, B and C. Most of the time two trends are much larger than the third one. Therefore the two big trends are not inclined to cooperate since they are competing for the top leadership. On the other hand, they try to set an agreement with the smaller trend. Accordingly let us assume A and B are the larger trends hostile to each other, while the smallest one is C.

On this basis the ABC configuration elects a C. It can result from a coalition with either A or B. Therefore, an A is elected only by either 2A or 3A, making the associated equation identical to the binomial form of Eq. (8.1). The same conditions hold for a B to be elected. Noting p, q and z as the respective probabilities of having an A, a B and a C elected, the equations at level $(n + 1)$ can be written as:

$$p_{n+1} = p_n^3 + 3p_n^2(1 - p_n), \tag{8.5}$$

$$q_{n+1} = q_n^3 + 3q_n^2(1 - q_n), \tag{8.6}$$

$$z_{n+1} = 1 - p_{n+1} - q_{n+1}, \tag{8.7}$$

where p_n, q_n and z_n are the proportions of elected persons A, B and C at level n. Both Eqs. (8.5) and (8.6) have the three fixed points 0, 1 and $\frac{1}{2}$ of which the last one is unstable. It is not the case for Eq. (8.7) whose dynamics results from those of both Eqs. (8.5) and (8.6).

In other words now, when overall support for both A and B are less than 50%, their respective supports become weaker while climbing the hierarchy level. As a mechanical consequence, C gets stronger and stronger proportions. Provided

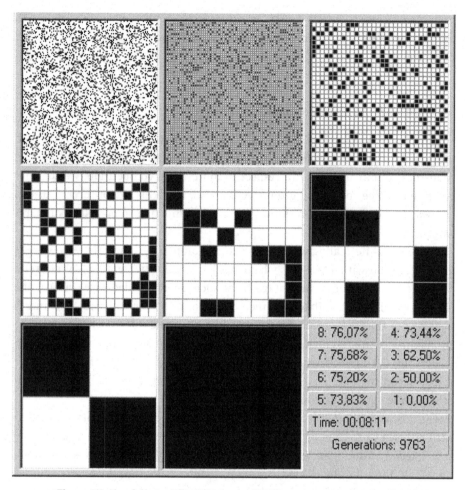

Figure 8.3 Simulation with 4096 persons. Written percentages are for the white representation at each level. At the bottom level there are 76.07% A (white) supporters. Now six levels are needed to get a black square (B) elected. The bottom-level B support (black) to hold on to power is at only 23.03%. The 'Time' and 'Generations' data should be ignored.

there exist enough levels, the presidency goes to C with certainty as soon as A and B score less than 50%.

In the case of there being only a few levels, C gets an increasing power weight-ing at higher hierarchical level. Let us illustrate such a process with some figures. Suppose A and B each hold 47% support with C scoring only 6%. A first level vot-ing this yields for A, B and C the outcomes 45%, 45% and 10% where these figures are obtained using respectively Eqs. (8.5), (8.6) and (8.7). A second voting level gives 40%, 40%, and 20%. At a third level the proportions become respectively 35%, 35% and 30%. A fourth level leads to 28%, 28% and 44%. Within four levels

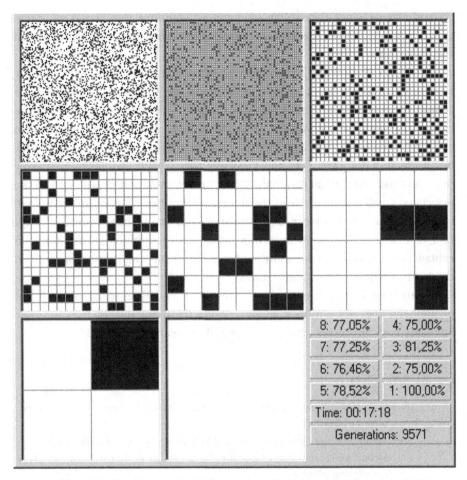

Figure 8.4 Simulation with 4096 persons. At the bottom level there are 77.05% A (white) supporters. Now the A trend (white) takes the presidency from the black (B) trend.

the ultra-minority trend C has been able to increase its proportion from 6% at the bottom level up to the leading proportion of 44%. Four additional levels yield the following series: 20%, 20%, 60%; 10%, 10%, 80%; 3%, 3%, 94% and 0%, 0%, 100%. The 6% trend gets the presidency with certainty within eight levels. Given only four levels C gets 30% of the elected persons below the president.

Conclusion

To conclude we comment on a possible application of the model to shed new light on the auto-collapse of Eastern European Communist parties during the last century. Up to this historical and drastic event, Communist parties seemed eternal. Once they collapsed many explanations were based on opportunistic change within the various organisations, with in addition the end of the Soviet Army threat.

Part of the explanation may be related to our hierarchical model. Communist organisations are based, at least in principle, on the concept of democratic centralism, which is nothing else than a tree-like hierarchy. Suppose then the critical threshold for gaining power was of order of 80%, as in our four-person cell case. We could then consider that the internal opposition to the orthodox leadership did grow a lot and massively over several decades to eventually reach and pass the critical threshold. Once the threshold was passed, we had the associated sudden taking over of the internal opposition. Therefore, the sudden collapse of Eastern European Communist parties would have been the result of a very long and solid phenomenon inside the Communist parties. Such an explanation does not oppose additional constraints but emphasises the internal mechanism within these organisations.

At this stage it is of importance to stress that modelling social and political phenomena does not aim to state an absolute truth but instead tries to single out some basic processes which are expected to be active in real life.

References

Bunde, A., Kropp, J. and Schellnhuber, H. J. (eds.) (2002). *The Science of Disasters*. New York: Springer-Verlag.

de Oliveira, S. M., de Oliveira, P. M. C. and Stauffer, D. (2000). *Non-Traditional Applications of Computational Statistical Physics: Sex, Money, War, and Computers*. New York: Springer-Verlag.

Galam, S. (1986). Majority rule, hierarchical structure and democratic totalitarianism. *J. Math. Psychol.* **30**, 426–434.

(1999). Le vote majoritaire est-il totalitaire? *Pour La Science, Hors série, Les Mathématiques Sociales*, July, 90–94.

(2000). Les réformes sont-elles impossibles? *Le Monde* 28 Mar., 18–19.

(2002). Minority opinion spreading in random geometry. *Eur. Phys. J. B* **25** (Rapid Note), 403–406.

Galam, S. and Wonczak, S. (2000). Dictatorship from majority rule voting. *Eur. Phys. J. B* **18**, 183–186.

Galam, S., Chopard, B., Masselot, A. and Droz, M. (1998). Competing species dynamics. *Eur. Phys. J. B* **4**, 529–531.

Ma, S.-K. (1976). *Modern Theory of Critical Phenomena*. Reading, MA: Benjamin Inc.

Pathria, R. K. (1972). *Statistical Mechanics*. Oxford: Pergamon Press.

9

Natural selection and complex systems: a complex interaction

DAVID SLOAN WILSON

Binghamton University

In their book *Darwinism Evolving*, Depew and Weber (1995) develop the thesis that evolutionary theory has been reformulated several times to keep pace with advances in knowledge about the physical world. Darwin's Newtonian formulation was replaced by a probabilistic formulation early in the twentieth century. According to Depew and Weber, the new science of complexity will force yet another formulation, which is taking place during our time.

This general thesis may well be correct but Depew and Weber's specific account of the relationship between evolution and complexity leaves much to be desired (Wilson, 1995). They largely accept the polemic view of Gould and Lewontin (1979) at face value, arguing that natural selection is far more constrained and adaptations less common than claimed by proponents of the so-called adaptationist programme. Complexity is viewed as something that stamps its own properties on organisms and resists the modifying effects of natural selection.

Depew and Weber are not alone in this view. Many complexity theorists and writers seem to parade under the banner 'Darwin is dead! Long live complexity!' The following passage by Kauffman (1993: 24) provides one example:

> In short, if selection is operating on systems with strongly self-organized properties that are typical of the ensemble being explored, then those properties simultaneously are the proper null hypothesis concerning what we would expect to find in the absence of selection and may be good predictors of what we will observe even in the presence of continuing selection. In brief, if selection can only

Self-Organisation and Evolution of Social Systems, ed. Charlotte K. Hemelrijk.
Published by Cambridge University Press. © Cambridge University Press 2005.

slightly displace evolutionary systems from the generic properties of the underlying ensembles, those properties will be widespread in organisms not because of selection, but despite it.

This view of evolution and complexity suffers from being – well, too simple. More of one means less of the other. Complexity replaces natural selection as an explanatory principle rather than interacting with it. In this chapter I will present three case studies that illustrate a more complex and synergistic relationship between natural selection and complex systems. The synergy occurs because complex systems have profound effects on phenotypic variation and heritability, the two basic ingredients of natural selection.

Case study 1: radical epistasis and the genotype–phenotype–fitness relationship

Many problems in evolutionary biology are represented by the metaphor of adaptive landscapes, which invokes an image of peaks of high fitness separated by valleys of low fitness. Natural selection is envisioned as a hill-climbing process that moves populations to the tops of local peaks but is unable to move from low peaks to higher peaks that are separated by valleys. In addition, this metaphor makes it difficult to see how a sexually reproducing population can occupy more than one peak, because when individuals that occupy two peaks mate with each other, their progeny will be intermediate and will occupy valleys of low fitness (with the exception of complete dominance in single-locus models). This metaphor has influenced thinking on speciation (Otte and Endler, 1989), genetic polymorphisms (e.g. Charlesworth and Charlesworth, 1975), recombination (Bell, 1982; Michod and Levin, 1988), and genetic load (Wallace, 1991).

I call the adaptive landscape a metaphor because it has proven difficult to model rigorously. Provine (1986) showed that at least three incompatible versions exist, in which a point on the landscape represents (a) the mean fitness of the population, (b) the fitness of a single genotype, or (c) the fitness of a single phenotype. Even Sewall Wright, the primary inventor of the concept, used all three versions without realising that they cannot be easily related to each other. To make matters worse, a variety of factors such as density- and frequency-dependent selection can turn the landscape into a seascape with undulating peaks and valleys and can prevent natural selection from climbing hills, which surely is an essential part of the metaphor!

The passage by Kauffman quoted above is based in part on a model in which each genotype in a multi-locus system is assigned a phenotype, which in turn is assigned a fitness. Complex (epistatic) genetic interactions are modelled by making the genotype–phenotype relationship non-additive. The ultimate in epistasis is for a single allele substitution at any locus to create a new phenotype that is completely independent of the old phenotype. Fortunately, this kind of radical epistasis is easy to model, by simply defining a phenotypic parameter space and randomly assigning a value to each genotype in a multi-locus system. Kauffman showed that this kind of radical epistasis creates a 'rugged' fitness landscape in which the population can easily become trapped on peaks of low fitness and cannot find its way to higher peaks. Furthermore, a population cannot occupy more than one peak because mating and recombination create maladaptive combinations.

Kauffman's model complicates the genotype–phenotype relationship but keeps the phenotype–fitness relationship simple by assigning a constant fitness value to each phenotype. In contrast, Wilson and Wells (1994) complicate the phenotype–fitness relationship by making fitness density-dependent. The phenotypic parameter space consists of six values (5–10) that represent either a two-peak landscape (phenotypes 5&6 and 9&10 are peaks of high fitness separated by 7&8 as a valley of low fitness), or a three-peak landscape (odd-numbered peaks separated by even-numbered valleys). Valley phenotypes have a constant low fitness (= zero in most simulations) but the fitness of peak phenotypes declines with the number of individuals occupying the peak. Negative density- and frequency-dependent forces are extremely common in nature so these assumptions are at least as realistic as assuming a constant fitness for each phenotype.

Given these assumptions, the maximally adaptive genetic system would create phenotypes that occupy the peaks in equal proportions and miss the valleys. Of course, this is not possible if mating is random and the genotype–phenotype relationship is additive. In this case, phenotypes that occupy different peaks mate and produce intermediate offspring that fall into the valleys. However, something quite remarkable happens when the genotype–phenotype relationship is made maximally epistatic. In this case, a subset of genotypes evolves that satisfies two criteria: (a) all genotypes occupy adaptive peaks, and (b) all genotypes give rise to each other by recombination. Thanks to epistasis, the progeny of two individuals, which are genetically intermediate by definition, need not be phenotypically intermediate, which makes it possible for the genetic system as a whole to occupy more than one peak while missing the valleys.

Because a multi-locus genetic system contains many genotypes, it potentially contains many subsets that satisfy the two criteria outlined above. A single genetic system can adapt itself to both a two-peak and a three-peak adaptive landscape merely by selecting different subsets of genotypes. It is even possible to 'train' a radically epistatic genetic system to adapt to long-term evolutionary change in which the adaptive landscape switches periodically between a two-peak and a three-peak landscape. In this case, a subset of genotypes can evolve that satisfies the two criteria for one landscape, and then satisfies the criteria for the other landscape with a single mutational change (unpublished simulations).

To summarise, the same radically epistatic genotype–phenotype relationship that constrains natural selection in Kauffman's model endows natural selection in our model with a remarkable ability to mould itself to multi-peak adaptive landscapes and swiftly adapt to long-term recurrent changes in the environment. The reason is obvious, if only in retrospect: a radically epistatic system allows almost any combination of phenotypes to be produced by a randomly mating subset of genotypes, without the production of intermediate forms that has always made evolution in multi-peak adaptive landscapes seem problematic.

Case study 2: group selection in humans and other animals

Natural selection within a single group is insensitive to the welfare of the group (Sober and Wilson, 1998). A solid citizen who behaves 'for the good of the group' will not increase its proportional representation within the group, and will even decline in frequency (ultimately going extinct) if providing the public good requires a private cost in time, energy or risk. Freeloaders are equally or more fit than solid citizens within groups. On the other hand, groups of solid citizens are more fit than groups of freeloaders. If there are many groups that vary in their proportions of solid citizens and freeloaders, the solid citizens can evolve by group-level selection despite their selective disadvantage within groups.

However, why should groups vary in their proportions of solid citizens and freeloaders? In the past, models that attempt to answer this question have been based on simple genotype–phenotype relationships, such as a single-locus model in which one allele codes for the solid citizen and the other codes for the freeloader. In this case, genetic and phenotypic variation become tightly linked to each other and the partitioning of variation within and among groups is determined straightforwardly by sampling error, declining precipitously with the number of individuals that independently colonise the groups. Since group selection requires variation among groups, the implication is that the importance of group selection declines rapidly with initial group size. These models contributed to the widespread rejection of group selection as an important evolutionary force in the 1960s. Few people questioned whether the verdict might have been based on the assumption of a simple genotype–phenotype relationship.

Subsequent research over the last few decades has amply shown that the rejection of group selection was premature. In the first place, real groups simply do not conform to expectations based on sampling error; they often vary greatly in their phenotypic properties, even when initiated by many individuals. In the second place, selection experiments reveal that phenotypic variation among groups is usually heritable, sometimes even more heritable than phenotypic variation among individuals within groups (Goodnight and Stevens, 1997). Group selection happens, in both nature and the laboratory, so why did the initial models fail so miserably to represent the real world?

The answer can be traced to the assumption of a simple genotype–phenotype relationship. More complex relationships can cause random genetic variation among groups to give rise to highly non-random phenotypic variation. There are many specific ways to do this but all of them can be understood as forms of sensitive dependence on initial conditions. A population of groups can be regarded as replicate biological systems that initially vary, if only at random. If the biological systems are complex in their genetic and social interactions, then the initial differences will not stay small but will provide the basis for larger differences – the 'butterfly effect' that is so well known for complex physical systems. Replicate complex systems are *expected* to vary, no matter how small their initial differences. We might wonder if the differences that develop are heritable, but we shouldn't be surprised by the raw fact of phenotypic variation among groups whose elements interact in a complex fashion, even if the initial variation is random.

I will provide one example of the decoupling of genetic and phenotypic variation, although many could be chosen. Wilson and Kniffin (1999) present a multilevel selection model in which genes code for social transmission rules rather than directly for behaviours. One rule is for conformity and can be stated formally as: 'converge upon a single behaviour, chosen randomly from the initial behaviours in the group'. If everyone in a group follows this rule, and if they enter the group exhibiting different behaviours, then all of them adopt a single behaviour chosen at random from the initial behaviours. There are a variety of specific mechanisms that might accomplish this but we need only focus on the final effect of behavioural uniformity within the group.

Now let's expand our scope to consider a large population of individuals who follow this rule. A fraction p behave like solid citizens while the remaining $(1 - p)$ behave like freeloaders. They form into many groups of size n at random. At first behavioural variation among groups follows the binomial distribution, but then the social transmission rule takes over and all groups become behaviourally uniform. Notice that the value of p has not changed in the total population because each group converges on one or the other behaviour at random, but the partitioning of the variation has changed dramatically. Initially most of the variation was within groups, whereas all of it becomes variation among groups thanks to the transmission rule. Of course, the new partitioning of variation is maximally favourable for group selection. The groups of solid citizens do well, the groups of freeloaders do poorly, there is no exploitation within groups, and so the differential fitness of groups increases the frequency of solid citizens (p) in the global population. If the groups break up and the individuals (or their progeny) form new groups at random, the transmission rule again eliminates variation within groups and maximises variation among groups, and the cycle repeats itself.

So far, this model shows how a population can be genetically uniform but phenotypically variable, and how large phenotypic differences among groups can develop even when the groups are randomly formed. However, it remains to show how this particular genetically encoded transmission rule can evolve in competition with other transmission rules. Wilson and Kniffin (1999) consider three rules in addition to the one already described: (a) a rule that resists changing its behaviour after entering a new group, (b) a rule that is biased toward becoming a solid citizen, and (c) a rule that is biased toward becoming a freeloader. A group formed by individuals with different transmission rules will not necessarily converge upon a single behaviour. Thus, there will be mixed groups in which freeloaders profit at the expense of the solid citizens. Nevertheless, the phenotypic variation among groups can still be non-random, despite the fact that the groups are randomly formed (Fig. 9.1). Moreover, the relationship between phenotypes and genotypes has become complex; a given genetic type can become either behavioural type. Even when the model includes 'recalcitrant' genotypes biased toward freeloading, this complex phenotype–genotype relationship can nevertheless favour the evolution of transmission rules that are not only conformist, but biased toward solid citizen behaviours. In more familiar terms, evolution in randomly formed groups can evolve the psychological disposition to figure out what's good for the group and make sure that everyone does it. More generally, this model is only one of many in which complex genotype–phenotype relationships make group selection a potent evolutionary force, even in groups initiated at random by large numbers of individuals.

Case study 3: ecosystem selection

The idea that entire ecosystems can evolve into adaptive units has been regarded as among the most extravagant claims of holistically minded biologists. Nevertheless, the same principles that I outlined in case study 2, which enable complex single-species systems to evolve into adaptive units, also apply to ecosystems consisting of multiple species interacting with each other and their abiotic environment.

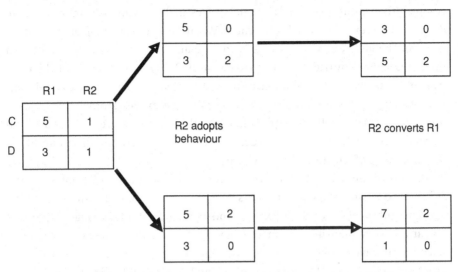

Figure 9.1 An interaction between behaviours (C and D) and transmission rules (R1 and R2) increases variation among groups. The transmission rules are assumed to be genetically encoded while the behaviours are acquired on the basis of the transmission rules. C and D are the behaviours 'cooperate' and 'defect' in a standard 'prisoner's dilemma' model. Individuals with transmission rule R1 retain their behaviour unless influenced by another transmission rule. Individuals with transmission rule R2 converge upon a single behaviour chosen at random from the initial behavioural composition of the group. In addition, each R2 individual is able to 'convert' a single R1 individual. The group starts with the initial composition of behaviours and transmission rules shown in the left-hand box and follows one of the two trajectories shown by the arrows, depending upon whether the R2s converge upon C or D. In a global population with many groups, the effect of these interactions is to decrease behavioural variation within groups and increase behavioural variation among groups, favouring the evolution of cooperation. From Wilson and Kniffin (1999).

Of course, ecosystems are vastly more complex than any single species. This is no argument against ecosystem selection, however, since the basic point of this essay is to show that complexity can *facilitate* the natural selection process. Consider the community of microbes, fungi and invertebrates that inhabit the root zone of plants. Each plant and its associated fauna can be regarded as a local ecosystem, whose members interact primarily among themselves and with the physical environment in the immediate vicinity of the plant. These local ecosystems will surely vary in their species composition and in the genetic composition of the component species. Even if the initial variation among ecosystems is slight, sensitive dependence is likely to magnify these differences, as described for single-species groups in case study 2. The fact that local ecosystems are more complex than local groups of a single species makes them even more likely to diverge on the basis of initial differences. Variation in the species/genetic composition of the local ecosystems is likely to have an effect on important ecosystem processes such as nutrient cycling, oxygen availability, modification of the physical substrate, and so on. Solid citizens and freeloaders are at least as relevant to ecosystem processes as to the dynamics of single-species groups. Local ecosystems that function well, perhaps by helping 'their' plant to grow vigorously and provide them with abundant resources, could then contribute differentially to the formation of future local ecosystems.

Simulation models (Wilson, 1992; Johnson and Boerlijst, 2002; Johnson and Seinen, 2002), laboratory experiments (Swenson et al., 2000a, b), and even a limited amount of field research (Wilson and Knollenberg, 1987) suggest that this scenario is fully plausible, no matter how far-fetched the concept of ecosystem selection may have appeared in the past. One key insight is that most ecological processes are local by their nature, which makes it possible to envision a large-scale ecosystem such as a forest as a population of many small local ecosystems. Once a population of ecosystems becomes plausible, complex interactions make variation among ecosystems almost inevitable. The ecosystems need not be separated by discrete boundaries. Simulation models show that even when species are placed on a uniform grid, such that each individual is at the centre of its neighbourhood, complex localized interactions result in spatial heterogeneity. If variation among patches on a landscape such as this has functional consequences, the stage is set for the successful patches to persist and spread at the expense of less successful patches.

The simulation model of Wilson (1992) illustrates how complex interactions can produce heritable variation at the level of multi-species communites. Local communities are colonised at random from a global pool of 10 species and interact for a period of time before dispersing back into the global pool. Species interactions are modelled with Lotka–Volterra equations and a three-dimensional matrix of interaction terms randomly and uniformly distributed between 0 and 2, where $a_{i,j,k}$ is the effect of species i on species j in the presence of species k. For every iteration of the difference equations, the three-dimensional matrix is collapsed into a two-dimensional matrix by averaging the 10 $a_{i,j}$ terms, weighted by the relative proportions of the 10 species in the patch. In this fashion, the pairwise species interactions depend upon the background composition of the local community.

These complex interactions cause initially random variation in the species composition of local communities to become highly non-random, as shown in Fig. 9.2. The upper graph shows the relative proportion of the 10 species in the global dispersal pool over the course of 21 cycles of local community

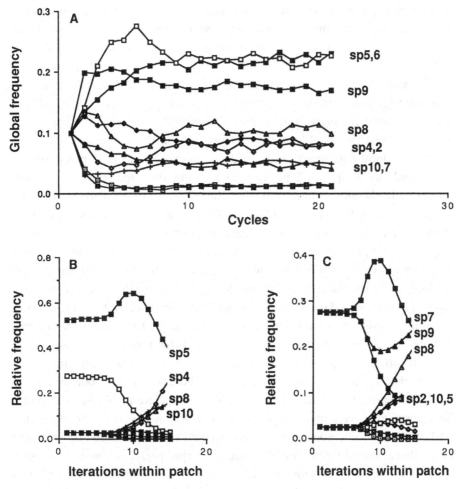

Figure 9.2 Community-level selection in a simulation model, in which local communities (patches) are colonised at random from a global pool of dispersers, and the species within each patch interact for a period of time before dispersing back into the global pool. The simulation is initiated with all species in equal frequency. (A) Changes in frequency in the global pool over 21 cycles of patch formation and dispersal; (B) and (C) the dynamics of two local patches. From Wilson (1992).

formation and dispersal. Community dynamics at the global scale looks fairly orderly and is governed by negative frequency-dependent selection. In other words, if any given species is displaced from its characteristic frequency, it will return to that frequency. The two lower graphs show the dynamics of a sample of local communities drawn at random from the global pool after it has reached its (rough) equilibrium. Community dynamics at the local scale is highly non-equilibrium, with the species composition embarking on different trajectories depending upon initial conditions. Nevertheless, the orderly dynamics at the global scale is produced by the combined non-equilibrium dynamics at the local scale.

The result of all this is that many species are maintained in the global pool and that local communities perpetually vary in their species composition. Now what happens if the local communities differentially go extinct and fail to contribute to the global pool (community-level selection)? For example, what happens when local communities are made to go extinct in direct proportion to the abundance of species 5 in Fig. 9.2? Not only does species 5 become less abundant in the global community, but the other species change their relative proportions as well, as shown in Fig. 9.3. The reason is that species 5 was abundant in some local communities and rare in others due to the presence of other species that supported or inhibited the growth of species 5. Community-level selection not only differentially removed species 5 but also its supporting cast (including species 4 and 19), while favouring the species that prevent species 5 from becoming abundant in the first place (including species 9, 2 and 7). Before community-level selection, we had a species that drove the entire local community extinct. After community-level selection, we have local communities that drive the offending species extinct or at least to low levels of abundance.

Empirically, the laboratory experiments of Swenson et al. (2000a, b) impressively demonstrate how the butterfly effect can operate in biological systems. Microcosms that were made as physically identical as possible were inoculated with millions of microbes from a single well-mixed source. Based on sampling error, there was negligible initial variation in the species composition of each microcosm, yet they became very different over a period of only a few days (which equals many microbial generations) and the differences had important consequences for ecosystem properties such plant growth, pH of the environment or degradation of a toxic compound (depending on the experiment). When these properties were used as a basis for selecting whole microcosms to colonise a new set of microcosms, there was a response to selection, demonstrating that the kind of phenotypic variation created by complex interactions can be heritable (Figs. 9.4 and 9.5).

One way to think about this experiment in terms of complex systems theory is to imagine a parameter space with $(S + 1)$ dimensions, where each axis represents the proportion of one species in an S-species ecosystem and the $(S + 1)$th axis measures the ecosystem property that serves as the basis for selection (e.g. pH of the medium). At the beginning of the experiment described above, the microcosms are represented by a small cloud of points in the parameter space, because they are nearly identical in their species composition except for

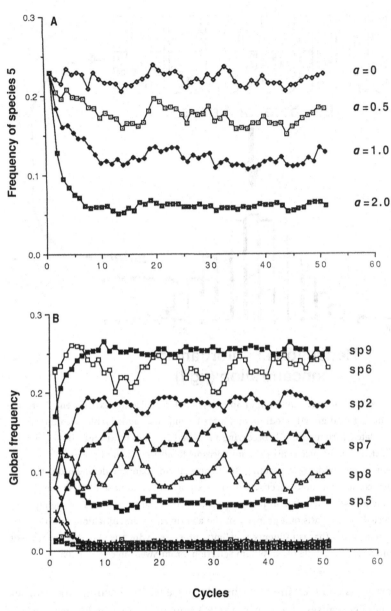

Figure 9.3 A continuation of Fig. 9.2, with the added factor that local communities go extinct in direct proportion to the abundance of species 5 just prior to dispersal. Note that species 5 is one of the most abundant species in the global community in Fig. 9.2, although its abundance varies at the patch level: (A) shows the change in the global frequency of species 5 as the intensity of extinction at the group level (governed by the a term) increases; (B) shows the frequency of all 10 species when $a = 2$, which can be compared to Fig. 9.2 when $a = 0$. Community-level selection changes the composition of the entire community, reducing not only species 5 but also its 'supporting cast'. See text and Wilson (1992) for more details.

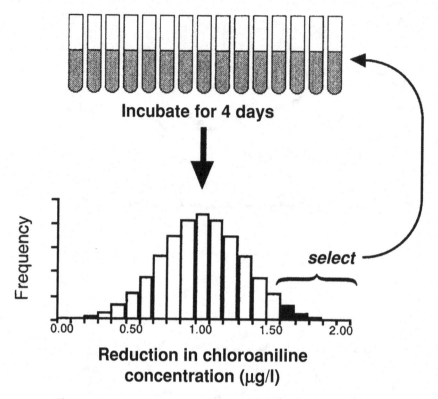

Incubate for 4 days

Reduction in chloroaniline concentration (μg/l)

Figure 9.4 Schematic diagram of an ecosystem-level selection experiment. Test tubes with microbial growth medium and a toxic compound added (chloroaniline) are inoculated with a naturally occurring microbial community from a single source. Sensitive dependence causes the microcosms to diverge in their species composition, with corresponding differences in chloroaniline degradation. The microcosms that most effectively degrade chloroaniline are used as 'parents' to create a new 'generation' of microcosms. Note that the microcosms are being selected on the basis of a property of the abiotic environment (chloroaniline concentration) that is influenced by biotic processes, which is why this experiment counts as an example of ecosystem selection. From Swenson *et al.* (2000a).

sampling error. As complex interactions take place within each microcosm, sensitive dependence causes them to embark upon separate trajectories and the cloud of points expands. To the degree that species composition influences the ecosystem property that serves as the basis for selection, variation will increase along the $(S + 1)$th axis as well. At the end of the first generation, the microcosms at one end of the distribution on the $(S + 1)$th axis are selected and used as the 'parents' which are mixed together and used to inoculate a second generation of microcosms. Variation at the beginning of the second generation is again represented by a small cloud of points, but the location of this cloud is

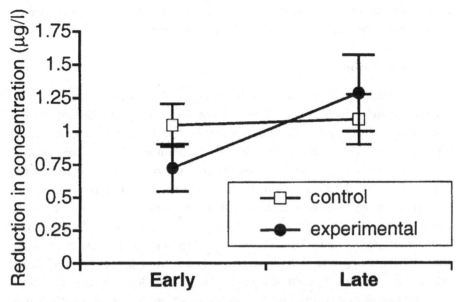

Figure 9.5 Response to selection in an ecosystem selection experiment. Four experimental lines selected for chloroaniline degradation increased their degradation ability on average, compared to four control lines in which the microcosms were selected at random. The average degradation ability of the experimental lines was (non-significantly) lower than the control lines at the beginning of the experiment by chance. From Swenson *et al.* (2000a).

different from that for the first generation. In this fashion, the experiment can be envisioned as a way of searching a very large parameter space for regions that create the phenotype being selected (e.g. high pH), similar to computer algorithms that use multiple agents to search large parameter spaces. However, regions of the parameter space that create the selected phenotype must also be locally stable for there to be a response to selection. In the absence of local stability, the ecosystems that were selected during one generation will give rise to ecosystems during the next generation that embark on trajectories of their own, with different effects on the ecosystem property that serves as the basis of selection. To summarise, if the parameter space includes regions that (a) create the phenotype being selected and (b) are locally stable, then the process of ecosystem selection can 'find' these regions. Switching back from the language of complex systems theory to the language of evolutionary theory, there will be phenotypic variation at the ecosystem level and some of it will be heritable. Notice that ecosystem selection can take place purely by changing species composition without any genetic changes in the component species. The local ecosystem has truly become the analogue of an organism and species have become the analogue of genes. However, the response to ecosystem selection can include genetic changes within species in addition to changes in species composition.

Conclusion

Scientific inquiry often begins at the simplest possible level and adds complexity only when needed. Thus it is not surprising that evolutionary and ecological models began by assuming simple interactions. However, the inadequacies of these assumptions are becoming apparent and further progress will require a greater appreciation of complexity in various forms. In this sense, Depew and Weber (1995) are right that a new formulation of evolutionary (and ecological) theory is in order. However, the new formulation will not merely assign a smaller role to natural selection and a larger role to the properties of complex systems that resist selection. Some resistant properties undoubtedly exist, but more important will be the properties of complex systems that facilitate natural selection. In each of my case studies, complex systems provided far more promising raw material for the sculpting action of natural selection than simple systems. How fitting that the relationship between natural selection and complexity is proving to be complex.

References

Bell, G. (1982). *The Masterpiece of Nature*. Berkeley, CA: University of California Press.

Charlesworth, D. and Charlesworth, B. (1975). Theoretical genetics of Batesian mimicry. I. Single-locus models. *J. Theoret. Biol.* **55**, 283–303.

Depew, D. J. and Weber, B. H. (1995). *Darwinism Evolving: Systems Dynamics and the Genealogy of Natural Selection*. Cambridge, MA: MIT Press.

Goodnight, C. J. and Stevens, L. (1997). Experimental studies of group selection: what do they tell us about group selection in nature? *Am. Naturalist* **150**, S59–S79.

Gould, S. J. and Lewontin, R. C. (1979). The spandrels of San Marco and the Panglossian paradigm: a critique of the adaptationist program. *Proc. Roy. Soc. London B* **205**, 581–598.

Johnson, C. R. and Boerlijst, M. C. (2002). Selection at the level of community: the importance of spatial structure. *Trends Ecol. Evol.* **17**, 83–90.

Johnson, C. R. and Seinen, I. (2002). Selection for restraint in competitive ability in spatial competition systems. *Proc. Roy. Soc. London B* **269**, 655–663.

Kauffman, S. A. (1993). *The Origins of Order*. Oxford: Oxford University Press.

Michod, R. E. and Levin, B. R. (eds.) (1988). *The Evolution of Sex*. Sunderland, MA: Sinauer Associates.

Otte, D. and Endler, J. A. (eds.) (1989). *Speciation and its Consequences*. Sunderland, MA: Sinauer Associates.

Provine, W. B. (1986). *Sewall Wright and Evolutionary Biology*. Chicago, IL: University of Chicago Press.

Sober, E. and Wilson, D. S. (1998). *Unto Others: The Evolution and Psychology of Unselfish Behavior*. Cambridge, MA: Harvard University Press.

Swenson, W., Arendt, J. and Wilson, D. S. (2000a). Artificial selection of microbial ecosystems for 3-chloroaniline biodegradation. *Envir. Microbiol.* **2**, 564–571.

Swenson, W., Wilson, D. S. and Elias, R. (2000b). Artificial ecosystem selection. *Proc. Natl Acad. Sci. USA* **97**, 9110–9114.

Wallace, B. (1991). *Fifty Years of Genetic Load: An Odyssey*. Ithaca, NY: Cornell University Press.

Wilson, D. S. (1992). The effect of complex interactions on variation between units of a metacommunity, with implications for biodiversity and higher levels of selection. *Ecology* **73**, 1984–2000.

(1995). Book review: *Darwinism Evolving: Systems Dynamics and the Genealogy of Natural Selection*. *Artif. Life* **2**, 261–267.

Wilson, D. S. and Kniffin, K. M. (1999). Multilevel selection and the social transmission of behavior. *Hum. Nature* **10**, 291–310.

Wilson, D. S. and Knollenberg, W. G. (1987). Adaptive indirect effects: the fitness of burying beetles with and without their phoretic mites. *Evol. Ecol.* **1**, 139–159.

Wilson, D. S. and Wells, A. (1994). Radical epistasis and the genotype–phenotype relationship. *Artif. Life* **2**, 117–128.

10

Interlocking of self-organisation and evolution

PAULIEN HOGEWEG

Utrecht University

Introduction

Organisms can cope with a variable environment in which various actions are called for in a variety of ways, e.g.:

- *'Red Queen' evolution.* Each individual performs the different types of actions with a pre-set frequency. There is some within-population/ species variation in these frequencies (i.e. it is a 'quasi-species'[1] rather than a monomorphic species). Because many variants are present in the population, changes in the environment will cause relatively rapid change in the population by selection of available genotypes of the quasi-species. In such a case the rate of change is fairly independent of mutation rate.
- *Frequency-dependent selection.* There are two or more subtypes in the population, each specialising on one or a subset of the actions. In contrast to the previous mode the within-population variation is not unimodal but multi-modal. Dependent on which actions are more in demand these subpopulations will increase/decrease. A clear-cut example is the distribution of the 'rover' and 'sitter' types in *Drosophila*, which do what the names suggest in foraging. The difference has been localized to

---

[1] The term 'quasi-species' is defined (Eigen and Schuster, 1979) as the distribution of genotypes produced by natural selection; this distribution corresponds to the eigenvector of the replication–mutation transition matrix in standard replicator equations.

Self-Organisation and Evolution of Social Systems, ed. Charlotte K. Hemelrijk.
Published by Cambridge University Press. © Cambridge University Press 2005.

two different alleles of a cGMP-dependent kinase gene which has plural effects, among which is a change in ion channels in the brain, ultimately leading to the two modes of exploiting food resources (Osborne *et al.*, 1997; Sokolowski, 1997; Renger *et al.*, 1999).

- *TODO-based behaviour.* TODO is an abbreviation for 'do what there is to do'. Each individual is capable of a variety of actions. Dependent on what is 'observed' in its local environment it 'chooses' its actions. In other words, individuals are conceived simply as stimulus response units. This contrasts with the artificial intelligence/artificial life models which describe 'optimal' action-planning. We have introduced the TODO principle as a powerful basis for self-organising processes. Because the performed actions change the environment, and the actions performed depend on the local environment, and because the locality differs per individual, TODO-based behaviour causes 'automatic' adaptation to the environment, as well as 'division of labour'. (We have shown in an unpublished study that TODO-based behaviour is sufficient to produce fine-grained age polyethism in bee colonies through the interaction with spatial pattern formation in the nest (Fig. 10.1).)

- *Self-reinforcing TODO.* Performing a certain action changes an internal state such that that action is more likely to be performed. Age-dependent polyethism, in particular with respect to foraging behaviour as seen in bees, seems in fact to belong to this category, and has been used as the basis for 'self-organising' division of labour in several models (e.g. Pacala *et al.*, 1996, Beshers *et al.*, 2001). Interestingly, it has been found recently (Ben-Shahar *et al.*, 2002) that the same cGMP-dependent kinase for which two alleles define the 'sitter' and 'rover' types of *Drosophila* defines the difference in forager and nurse bees. In the latter case the differentiation is not due to two alleles, but due to over-expression of the protein in the foragers relative to the nurse bees. Thus the same mechanism seems to define 'outgoing' vs. 'homely' behaviour in these phylogenetically distant insects, but the regulation differs: in *Drosophila* it depends on an evolutionary mechanism, whereas in bees it depends on an environmentally or interactionally (see below) induced physiological change.

Much work on self-organising behaviour which is done within this paradigm focuses on interactions between individuals within a conspecific group. In particular social insects, but also mammalian, in particular primate, 'social' groups (e.g. Hemelrijk, 1998, 1999, 2000a, b) have been studied in this way. This research has highlighted the rich repertoire of side effects that simple interactions, e.g. dominance

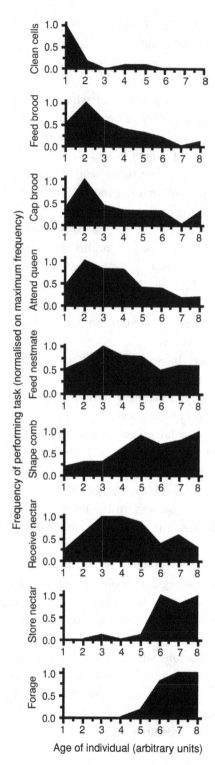

Figure 10.1 Division of labour in a beehive. Based on the observations of Seeley (1982) and Seeley and Kolmes (1991) that (1) different actions are performed in different parts of the nest, (2) different age groups perform preferentially different actions and (3) the within-hive age polyethism is only apparent in large nests, we developed a TODO-based model in which the behavioural repertoire of each bee included all possible actions. The actions were triggered by the local environment, and changed the local environment. This appeared to be suffcient to produce both the spatial nest structure and the age polyethism. The picture shows the behavioural profile of the relative frequency of the actions and is strikingly similar to the profiles in Seeley (1982). For other models on comb self-structuring, see Camazine et al. (2001: ch. 16).

interactions, can have. We have coined the term 'socio-informatic processes' for such interactions, which can be exploited as a means of obtaining information about the environment in an indirect manner. Examples of the latter include the well-known trail-laying strategy for finding food in ants (see Camazine *et al.*, 2001: ch. 13), a proposed socially regulated 'clock' in bumble-bees by which the end of the season can be 'perceived' (Hogeweg and Hesper, 1983, 1985), and (even with a minimum of reinforcement) the aggregation of slime moulds, by which light and temperature gradients can be perceived in the multicellular slug stage (Marée *et al.*, 1999a, b), as opposed to the unicellular stage.

- *'Environmental engineering'*. Variation in the environment is controlled, i.e. is made less variable or more predictable, by moulding the environment. In fact extensive moulding of the environment can be achieved by TODO-based mechanisms and at the same time this phenomenon provides the power of the TODO-based mechanisms in moulding behaviour patterns. However, it is also a powerful mechanism in an evolutionary context, providing selection pressures over a variety of timescales, leading to counter-intuitive outcomes of Darwinian evolution (as discussed below).

This list highlights how behavioural variation can be regulated either by evolutionary processes, by stimulus response and/or by physiological adaptation. Note that the variation in the behaviour, and the mode by which the switching is achieved, appear to be independent. Indeed the intricate relationship between 'evolutionary adaptation' and 'physiological adaptation' (possibly mediated by individual interactions) is highlighted in recent experimental research. The *Drosophila*/bee case mentioned above is one example. Another example, from yeast, is the demonstration that a small number of mutations can give rise to massive changes in gene expression by mediation of gene regulation networks – and therefore produce variants which phenotypically resemble alternate phenotypes produced by physiological adaptation (Ferea *et al.*, 1999).

Nevertheless, most research on behavioural adaptation and differentiation is targeted at the different classes of mechanisms in isolation. In particular, interactions between evolutionary and self-organisation processes are not considered, even when the existence of the interactions are acknowledged (e.g Camazine *et al.*, 2001). I can think of two reasons for this: (1) separation of timescales is a method often used for model simplification, and appears at first sight to be appropriate; (2) there appears to be a motivational gap between those who like to emphasise that the properties of the basic units under consideration (organisms) change over time, and those who like to emphasise that the basic units (rules) may remain constant and yet produce behavioural change at another level. In the latter case the basic framework of modelling dynamical systems in terms of parameters and variables can be retained.

In contrast, the main argument in this chapter will be that it is essential to study self-organisation and evolution in consort. First I show that the timescale argument is not valid. Evolution is not something that 'happened long ago and far away' in order to fix the parameters of the system (model) under consideration. Neither is what happens on a short timescale (ecologically or within a lifetime) merely 'noise' for evolutionary processes. Next I will focus on two aspects of the concurrence of self-organisation and evolution, namely (1) how, in an eco-evolutionary context, spatial self-organisation generates new levels of selection, and thereby directs evolution of the basic replicating entities into unexpected directions, and (2) how cellular self-organisation occurs as a consequence of the interlocking of intra- and intercellular dynamics, and how this causes genomic self-organisation, and, in a sense, 'directed' evolution.

Interlocking ecological and evolutionary timescales

In this section I review a very simple model (van der Laan and Hogeweg, 1995) which demonstrates the potential interlocking of evolutionary and ecological timescales, even when the prior defined timescales of mutation and replication are very different (up to five orders of magnitude). The ecological dynamics is a simple oscillatory Lotka–Volterra-like predator–prey model. The evolutionary dynamics is defined on a single (circular) phenotype axis for both the predator and the prey. We can think of this phenotype axis as 'time of the day active'. There is global competition between all prey variants. In contrast predator variants interact only with 'corresponding' prey variants, i.e. they catch and eat prey variants with a Gaussian probability round their corresponding position on the prey phenotype axis. For the results reported below, the initial conditions are not important; we used either one predator and one prey variant on top of each other, or distributed predator and prey variants with a uniform distribution over the phenotype axis.

The dynamics of this model leads for certain widths of the Gaussian distribution to an eco-evolutionary attractor in which there are two quasi-(sub)species of predator and prey each. This 'speciation' process can be seen as self-organisation in phenotype space (compare Turing patterns) (Fig. 10.2). We note the following properties of this attractor:

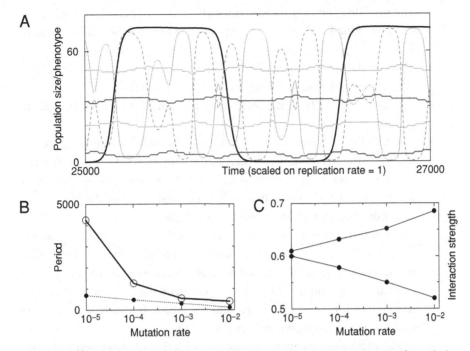

Figure 10.2 Ecological vs. eco-evolutionary timescales. (A) Time course of population size and average phenotypes. The thick black line indicates the oscillations in population size of the predators in the 'ecological' model (one predator); the dotted lines those of two predator subspecies in the eco-evolutionary model: they oscillate chaotically and in antiphase. Replication rate = 1, mutation rate = 0.0001. In the same graph phenotypic oscillations are drawn. In that case the vertical axis represents position on phenotype axis (0–60; periodic boundary conditions). The thin lines depict the low-amplitude oscillations representing the evolutionary 'wiggles' in phenotype space (light, prey; dark, predator) of the average location of the sub-quasi-species on the eco-evolutionary model. (B) Timescale vs. mutation rate $(10^{-5}-10^{-2})$: the lower the mutation rate, the more its inclusion speeds up the dynamics of the system. (C) Relative specialisation of the subspecies. The vertical axis represents interaction strength between predators and prey. The upper line is the average interaction strength between the predator subspecies and the prey subspecies nearest to them in phenotype space, and the lower line that for the other prey species. The divergence of the lines shows that almost no specialisation is present at low mutation rates, but that stronger specialisation occurs at higher mutation rates.

- The predator and prey quasi-species alternate in phenotype space. Thus each predator quasi-species can exploit each prey species, although there is a slight specialisation.
- The population numbers of the subspecies oscillate in counter-phase; the total population numbers are close to constant.
- The evolutionary dynamics oscillates with a small amplitude (wiggle) in phenotype space.
- The stability of the attractor depends on the combination of ecological and evolutionary dynamics. When mutation rate is set to zero (after the attractor is reached) the system collapses to at most a single predator and a single prey variant. Indeed it is the instability of the 'ecological' situation that drives the evolutionary 'wiggle'.
- An alternative way of defining the ecological dynamics of the system is by extracting the average interaction parameters between the two predator and two prey species over an integer number (e.g. 20) of periods. The resulting four coupled difference equations define a persistent ecological system for these precise parameter values, but only if we assume that arbitrary small populations are viable.
- In Fig. 10.2A we compare the period of oscillation of the eco-evolutionary system (thin lines) and the above-defined ecological system (thick lines). *The period is much longer in the ecology-only case.* This effect becomes even stronger when the intrinsic timescales of replication and mutation are more separated. This is shown in Fig. 10.2B: decreasing the mutation rate, while keeping the birth/death rate constant, increases the period of the oscillation of the ecological (four-difference equation) model much more than that of the full eco-evolutionary model. As shown in Fig. 10.2C, increasing the mutation rate leads in the eco-evolutionary model to more specialisation of the predators, which influences the timescale.

By adhering to the conventional ecological modelling framework, this example highlights the impact of 'just' adding mutations. The reversal of the effective ecological and evolutionary timescale (i.e. period of the wiggles) comes from both ends: the extremely long ecological timescales that occur in multi-species population interactions, and the short timescale over which evolution operates despite low mutation rates because of the maintenance of variation in the (sub)populations, i.e. dealing with quasi-species instead of monomorphic species; thus one does not have to 'wait 'for the appropriate mutation to occur.

It is interesting to note that VanderMeer (1993) studied the two predator–two prey system with weak specialisation of the predators and showed that very complicated and diverse chaotic dynamics can occur. Adding mutations channels the system into the weakly chaotic attractors shown here, which have faster dynamics and smaller amplitude fluctuations. Indeed this example suggests that *ongoing* evolutionary dynamics may be *a* solution to the long-standing problem of the stability and persistence of relatively diverse ecosystems (space being another strong candidate).

We conclude that studying eco-evolutionary dynamics is to be preferred above studying ecological dynamics and evolutionary dynamics separately. Especially in larger systems, where full parameter sweeps are impossible (and non-informative) including evolution might in fact make it easier to study the system as as it indicates which parameter choices are relevant (see also Hogeweg, 1998). We conjecture that similarly a combined study of non-inherited behavioural differentiation and evolution should be attempted. Current work on learning/ evolution of what to eat (van der Post and Hogeweg, 2004; W. Zuidema, unpubl. data) are attempts to do so.

Self-organisation and multi-level evolution

Classical population genetic theory has not tackled the intriguing question how an increase in complexity can evolve. Maynard Smith and Száthmary (1995) point out this fact, and conclude that major transitions have occurred which increased the complexity of living systems. These major transitions involve the generation of new levels of selection: replicators which are initially self-sufficient become part of coordinated larger units, which become new levels of selection. They document this process in early evolution, i.e. from self-replicating molecules to vesicles, and in later stages, e.g. the transition from prokaryotic to eukaryotic cells, from unicellular to multicellular organisms and from solitary insects to social insects.

Tackling the same problem from a different angle, in which we do not examine what *did* happen on earth, but what *does* happen in simple constructive models of eco-evolutionary dynamics, we found that new levels of selection occur automatically through self-organisation. The dynamics of the self-organised higher-level entities enslave the evolutionary fate of the basic entities that generate them. We demonstrated this first in the Hypercycle model of Eigen and Schuster (1979) of pre-biotic evolution (Boerlijst and Hogeweg, 1991a, b) The spiral patterns which form in spatial versions of the model cause a reversal of virtually all evolutionary properties of the self-replicating molecules with cyclic catalysis. For example, 'cheaters' ('parasites') can temporarily invade the system, but do not destroy it; there is positive selection for giving catalysis (altruism); and there even is positive selection for early death. All these properties can be understood in terms of (well-known) properties of spiral dynamics. In these early studies we adhered to the convention of separating ecological and evolutionary timescales, and studied the fate of invading mutants in an ecologically stabilized system. Here we will examine some related, later work which does not assume such timescale separation, and thereby highlights the mutual influence of self-organisation and evolution.

Evolutionary reinforcement of self-organised spatial patterns

As in the previous section we use a simple ecological model to highlight the influence of just two additions: space and mutations. Savill *et al.* (1997) used a coupled lattice map model based on Nicholson Baily host–parasitoid dynamics. Coupling is through migration of both the host and parasitoid. The host migrates randomly. The parasitoid may make a choice based on host density in adjacent squares. This preference has the form

$$p_i = kH_i / \sum (H_j)^b$$

where H denotes the host density, the sum is taken over the neighbouring patches (j) of patch i, k is a scaling constant and b is the evolving parameter which determines the degree of directed migration. If $b = 0$ unbiased diffusion occurs; if $b = 1$ the parasitoids spread proportional to host density in the neighbouring patches.

The population interactions lead for a wide range of parameters to spatial patterns which consist of a mixture of regions of spiral waves and regions of chaotic waves. This type of spatial pattern is known from the generic Complex Ginsburg Landau equation. In the eco-evolutionary context it means that there are three levels of selection: (1) the basic replicators, i.e. the host and the parasitoid, (2) the spiral waves whose dynamics is well understood, and (3) the (competing) regions of spiral patterns and chaotic waves of which the dynamics is much less well understood. Evolution, in this case of the diffusion bias towards hosts of the parasitoids, and the spatial self-organisation interlock in a complicated way. We observe:

- Parasitoids with the highest b value (i.e. those that migrate preferentially towards high host densities) have the highest short-term fitness, wherever they occur in the field.
- Nevertheless, within spirals the majority of parasitoids retain relatively low b values (0.5–0.9). In the chaotic regions the values stabilise at $b = 1.4$.
- The relative areas occupied by spirals and chaotic regions depend on the b parameter. When we study the ecological rather than the eco-evolutionary system (i.e. if we keep the value of b constant) spiral

regions dominate for low values of b, and chaotic regions for high values. Thus we see that the direction of evolution of the b parameter is such that it favours the type of pattern in which it finds itself.

- The evolution of low b values within spirals is due to the spiral dynamics: within spirals in the long term all offspring comes from the core, i.e. the spiral core serves as a kind of 'germ line'. Parasitoids with low b values are of course more likely to remain in the core.

- The b values in spirals, however, do not evolve to the lowest possible values and retain high variability due to spiral competition. Spirals with parasitoids with higher b values rotate faster and out-compete slower rotating spirals.

- Due to the evolution of the b parameter spirals display a definite 'life history'. They are generated on the edge of spiral regions and chaotic regions, and have initially high b values (which are selected in chaotic regions). Because of the evolution to low b values in the core, their rotation speed slows down with age. Because of between-spiral competition, their domain shrinks, and finally they die.

- The final outcome of the eco-evolutionary interactions depends on the competition between spiral regions and chaotic regions (i.e. the highest level of selection). At the edge between the regions new spirals are born. If birth rate exceeds death rate, spiral regions grow, otherwise chaotic regions grow; the evolution of the b parameter follows.

This rich dynamics of three levels of selection exemplifies clearly the 'environmental engineering' by the interacting individuals. They create higher-level entities with their own dynamics and 'life history'. The evolution of the basic entities (the 'only' entities as far as the model formulation is concerned) becomes enslaved to the dynamics of the higher-level entities they create. One of the consequences is the shift in timescales: those that have low short-term fitness in all locations may yet 'inherit the earth' (Fig. 10.3).

Similar effects have now been demonstrated in a variety of systems (e.g. Savill and Hogeweg, 1997; Johnson and Boerlijst, 2002; Johnson and Seinen, 2002). Savill and Hogeweg (1997) used a spatial version of the model discussed in the previous section, which illustrates nicely the interlocking of pattern formation in phenotype space and in space–space. Note that the phenomena discussed here in relation to spiral wave patterns do not depend on this particular type of spatial pattern but is rather a property of spatial pattern formation in general. Because the dynamics of spiral waves is well characterised, we can analyse in that case in detail the contribution of spatial pattern formation to the evolutionary outcome. In the examples below, the spatial pattern formation is chaotic

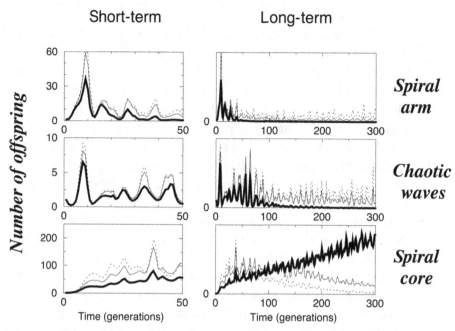

Figure 10.3 Short-term and long-term fitness. The left panels show short-term fitness (50 generations) and the right panels long-term fitness (300 generations) at three different locations in space (top: spiral arm, middle: chaotic region, bottom: spiral core.) The vertical axis gives average number of offspring per individual parasite with different aggregation tendency towards their host: thick line low, thin line intermediate and dotted line high aggregation tendency. At all locations high aggregation tendency gives the highest number of offspring over a time-slice of 50 generations. Nevertheless in the long run the fitness of parasites with the lowest aggregation tendency is the highest overall, as the number of offspring emanating from the core is much larger than from any other area. Note that this is the case in the eco-evolutionary attractor of the system, i.e. for any time-slice of 50 vs. 300 generations.

and not well characterisable. In that case its essential role is demonstrated by comparing the behaviour of the system with and without allowing spatial pattern formation.

Population-based vs. individual-based diversity

In the previous section the simple ecological models did not allow versatile behaviour of the basic entities. Here we look at a model in which a 'behavioural repertoire' can be built up during evolution, and study under which circumstances this will happen. Another difference from the previous section is that we define a priori two levels of selection; but as in the previous section we allow spatial pattern formation and therewith the generation of new levels of selection. The two a priori defined levels are bacteria and plasmids. The plasmids contain toxicity/immunity pairs of genes and determine the interaction among bacteria. Two versions of the system were studied, one modelling colicines (Pagie and Hogeweg, 1999, Czaran *et al.*, 2002), and one modelling restriction enzymes (Pagie and Hogeweg, 2000a, b). In the latter case viruses were included in the model as well.

For both systems a large variety of plasmids exist in nature. However in models in which spatial pattern formation is not possible the coexistence of all the variants cannot be understood. In the spatial models, however, where bacteria compete locally, there are two distinct ways in which plasmid diversity evolves and persists, i.e.:

- The bacteria diversify into many variants; each variant contains only a few plasmids. We call this mode population-based diversity.
- All bacteria contain almost all plasmids. We call this mode individual-based diversity.
- In the colicine system there is a phase transition between these two modes, dependent on cost of maintaining plasmids.
- Higher cost of carrying colicine plasmids decreases the population density of bacteria in the individual-based mode but, counter-intuitively, the opposite is true in the population-based mode where higher cost to the bacteria slightly increases population density.
- In the restriction enzyme system the modes are alternate attractors which both exist for a large overlapping parameter range.
- Here the population-based diversity benefits the bacterial population strongly: much higher population densities are maintained than in the individual-based mode. The bacteria carry different restriction enzymes and therewith accomplish a type of 'division of labour' to fight the viruses. This is very effective because the viruses obtain resistance only to a subset of the restriction enzymes and are killed off by the others.
- In contrast the 'clever' individuals in the individual-based mode benefit mainly the plasmids: the viruses become resistant to all restriction enzymes and kill off the bacteria. This leads to waves of infection and escape similar to those known from many host–parasitoid systems.

The various types of plasmids do not interfere within the bacteria, i.e. they add capabilities to the bacteria in modular form. Such modularity allows bacteria to share plasmids across species as is the case in antibiotic resistance. Similarly, TODO-like rules are also assumed to be modular. However, both TODO-like rules and plasmids interfere indirectly via the environment; this indirect interaction leads to the interesting and often counter-intuitive behaviour of the model. The models reviewed so far show that collecting more and more capabilities can evolve – but whether it indeed does so depends on the evolutionary dynamics rather than on the direct fitness it conveys. Many genetic systems are, however, not modular and many internal side effects occur by altering (the expression of) a gene as discussed above. In the next section we consider such internally coupled systems.

Genomic self-organisation and mutational 'priming'

The concept 'adaptive mutation' is, partly for historical reasons, a taboo in evolutionary theory. Discussions about the concept often get bogged down in statistics of insufficient data. More interestingly, genomic studies suggest both mutational and gene regulation mechanisms which could yield equivalent phenomena within the framework of Darwinian evolutionary theory. Mutational mechanisms include the repair mechanisms which may be switched on and off, and which may affect certain genes more or less (we will not consider those here). Moreover, it seems feasible that gene regulation networks are such that a variety of mutations cause them to switch between 'adaptive' attractors. The experimental results of Ferea et al. (1999), mentioned above, which show that a few mutations cause a massive change in gene expression, an increase in fitness, and a switch from one metabolic pathway to another, suggest such an attractor switching mechanism, that can be triggered either by physiological mechanisms, or, in other circumstances, by evolution. On a different scale, recent phylogenetic studies indicate that 'major morphological inventions' may not be monophyletic, but reoccur several times within certain lineages (and never outside these lineages). Similarly niche filling differentiation (speciation) can re-evolve on islands (or in lakes) repeatedly, even starting from different 'seeding' species/ecotypes (Givnish and Sytsma, 1997).

Although such results are compatible with a random mutation/selection mechanism the repeated convergence to a similar set of very divergent phenotypes in short evolutionary time suggests that within these species these phenotypes are 'easy' to reach and only a few mutations apart.

Here we will discuss model studies, based solely on random mutations and selection, which, through genomic self-organisation, exhibit phenotypic bias of the outcome of the (random) mutations. The three studies we review tackle this question from different angles, namely from the viewpoint of the dynamics of metabolic/genetic networks, from the viewpoint of co-evolution, and from the viewpoint of morphogenesis.

Evolutionary consequences of intracellular attractor dynamics

In a series of interesting papers, Kaneko and co-workers (e.g. Kaneko and Yomo, 1997, 2000, 2002; Furusawa and Kaneko, 2000, 2001) have examined, from a dynamical systems standpoint, what the consequences are of oscillatory and chaotic intracellular dynamics. To what extend such dynamics occur in cells is not well known, but many specific examples have been described (see for theoretical work the book of Goldbeter (1996)) and on general theoretical grounds one should expect such dynamics to occur in large, coupled networks. Indeed a certain percentage of randomly coupled metabolic networks do exhibit such oscillatory behaviour. Selecting those, or imposing such dynamics in the model formulation in the form of coupled sinusoidal functions, the authors studied growing populations of such cells, which share nutrients in the environment. They describe the following generic behaviour:

- Initially identical cells will differentiate into two or more well-defined attractors, i.e. cell types.
- An approximately fixed ratio of the different cell types is automatically maintained, even after disturbance (e.g. killing off part of the cells).
- The differentiation in a sense optimises growth rate of the population as a whole, but some cell types represent a kind of 'rest' state, and have a low growth rate.
- The differentiated cell types usually contain fewer different molecules in non-zero concentration than the 'stem' cell.

Thus this model produces as a generic property a 'division of labour' which is environmentally induced and optimises the growth of the entire population. Moreover, this happens notwithstanding the fact that the perceived environment is identical for all cells. This process is called 'isologous differentiation' by the authors and they cite experiments on E. coli which indicate that such differentiation indeed occurs in a genetically identical population. They also compare the model with stem cell differentiation within an individual.

To study evolutionary dynamics within this framework of self-organised dynamics, three extensions are needed: (a) competition between the cells (i.e. total population size is held approximately constant), (b) differential cell division and (c) mutation of the parameters. Differential cell division is due to differential accumulation of biomass, and can be modelled as the number of cycles of any of the attractors. After cell division the cell state is strongly perturbed, i.e. there is no phenotypic inheritance. The following is observed (Kaneko and Yomo, 2000, 2002):

- The cells first exhibit phenotypic differentiation as described above.
- During this stage phenotype is not inherited, and cells can re-differentiate into each other.
- The differentiated cell types maintain each other: each cannot exist without the other.
- Genetic differentiation occurs later; depending on the differentiated phenotype different mutations are advantageous.
- Thus the initially genetically identical cell lines diverge and do this in such a way that the domain of attraction of the attractor in which they find themselves is enlarged.
- Eventually genetic differentiation leads to inheritance of the phenotype because that phenotype becomes the only attractor of the network.
- This pathway allows for sympatric speciation in sexual populations because of the absence of 'viable' intermediates, i.e. for intermediate parameters the cells do not grow.
- After speciation the self-maintaining properties are lost; the two sub-populations in the end only compete, and one will out-compete the other.

Thus this system exhibits a 'phenotype first' scenario of speciation, within a strict Darwinian selection framework. Moreover, evolution is predictable from the internal dynamics of the system, i.e. it follows the available alternative attractors.

Co-evolution and mutational vs. computational modes of adaptation

In the previous model the evolutionary dynamics leads, in the terminology introduced above (pp. 176–178), to population-based diversity and loses its versatility to switch attractors. In this section we again take up the problem under which circumstances behavioural versatility (individual-based diversity) will evolve. We will contrast 'behavioural versatility', i.e. the ability to generate appropriate responses to different environments by attractor switching, with 'evolutionary versatility', i.e. the ability to evolve easily towards a higher fitness. The former can be called a 'computational' mode of adaptation as the appropriate response is 'computed' on the basis of the environmental input, whereas the latter can be called 'mutational' adaptation, i.e. the 'useful' mutations occur frequently enough and are selected by the environment. In contrast to the earlier model (see pp. 176–178) we now include a richer internal dynamics, and focus on the recognition part of a TODO mechanism: i.e. in order to do what there is to do, one has to recognise what there is to do.

Density classification by a cellular automaton has been extensively used as a paradigm system of 'emergent computation' (Crutchfield and Mitchell, 1995). Given an initial condition of 0s and 1s, the cellular automaton has to transform this initial configuration to all 0s in the case of a majority of 0s, and to all 1s when there is a majority of 1s. Perfect classification is not possible, but several rules having a >80% accuracy have been found. Several authors have used genetic algorithms to find such a 'good' rule, with mixed success (see Pagie and Mitchell, 2002) Here we consider this system, and its evolution, as a test-bed for the evolution of alternate 'adaptive strategies', i.e. adaption by 'computation' (leading to the 'appropriate' action) and adaptation by mutational attractor switching.

We use two populations, one of cellular automaton rules, i.e. the 'classifiers' and one of 'initial conditions' (of the cellular automata) which co-evolve. We again use a spatial set-up in which interaction is confined to neighbouring squares only. Fitness of the classifiers depends on the number of correct classifications, fitness of initial conditions depends on the number of false classifications (i.e. not being classified correctly conveys fitness to the initial conditions). The mutational bias of the initial conditions to the hardest cases (i.e. close to 50% 0s and 1s) is compensated by weighting fitness such that (mis)classification of easiest cases contributes most to fitness (for further details see Pagie (1999) and Pagie and Hogeweg (2000a, b)).

The outcome of the model depends on spatial pattern formation. In the case in which spatial pattern formation is prevented by global mixing between every time-step, 'mutational adaptation' evolves. Without mixing, spatial pattern formation occurs, and 'computational adaptation' evolves. In the case of 'computational adaptation' we see:

- The population of initial conditions occurs in two variable subpopulations with densities of between 40% and <50% and between >50% and 60% respectively.
- These subpopulations move as chaotic waves through the space.
- Classifiers classify quite well, both with respect to the available initial conditions, and with respect to externally provided, non-co-evolved, initial conditions, and also those with a density close to 50%, i.e. the hardest cases which are seldom 'seen'.
- Initial conditions are, in relation to their density, relatively hard to classify, i.e. they try to 'fool' classifiers by e.g. large blocks of 1s while there is, nevertheless, a majority of 0s.

- Classifiers use a sophisticated strategy for classification, the so-called 'particle-based' strategy, in which long-range communication within the cellular automata is used to determine the density, and are therefore less easily 'fooled'.
- Thus, there is an ongoing race between initial conditions and classifiers. The former can only change by mutation, but the latter are versatile TODO-ers which perform sophisticated computation on their input, but have to change evolutionarily as well to cope with the evolving initial conditions.

In the case of 'mutational adaptation' we see:

- At most times both the populations of classifiers and initial conditions are 'phenotypically converged', i.e. the initial conditions all have either a majority of 0s or a majority of 1s, and the classifiers recognise them correctly.
- Genetically both population are, however, diverse.
- The classifiers are 'single-minded', i.e. they classify all initial conditions, independent of density.
- Once in a while, an initial condition switches to the other majority class, and attains high fitness, taking over the population in a short time.
- Soon, however, the classifiers again achieve correct classification of all existing initial conditions: they remain 'single-minded' (classifying all initial conditions in the same way) but in the opposite way from before.

The rapid switching appears to be a side effect of the evolutionary scenario, and requires a special 'single-mindedness' which is retained by the recognition system (i.e. the cellular automaton rule) of a small subpopulation of the classifiers. In these classifiers a single mutation can switch the recognition system between the all-0 and the all-1 attractor. This despite the fact that most random cellular automaton rules are 'undetermined' relative to the density classification task, i.e. reach neither of the attractors for all or most initial conditions. In other words, evolutionary adaptation is optimised in this mutational adaptation attractor.

It is interesting to note that the average fitness of classifiers (and hence of the initial conditions) is very similar in both evolutionary attractors. In other words the mutational priming that occurs for the single-minded critters which evolve in the mixed case is as effective as the sophisticated computation which evolves in the non-mixed case (Fig. 10.4). Note that the mixing is the only difference between the models and that again the spatial patterning affects the evolutionary outcome profoundly.

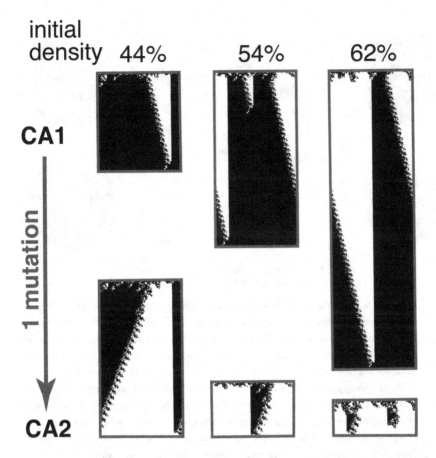

Figure 10.4 Evolutionary adaptation and mutational priming. Evolved classifiers without spatial pattern formation. The picture shows the transformation of the initial condition by the cellular automation (CA) rule until a homogeneous final state is reached. Black pixels denote state 0, white pixels state 1. Three initial conditions, with density of 44%, 54% and 62% of 1 are processed by two classifiers (upper and lower panels), which differ by just one mutation. The one mutation switches the attractor or the system from all-0 to all-1. The attractor is reached independent of initial conditions, i.e. the classifiers do not classify, but the mutation switches the response of the classifiers to all initial conditions. Because of convergence of the initial condition population such a switchable 'single-minded' response conveys high fitness.

Mosaic-like evolution and morphogenesis

In this section we revisit in another context the themes of the previous two subsections, i.e. the 'phenotype-first' effect and the 'mutational priming' of (apparently) large-scale phenotypic changes. We do so in a model of morphogenesis, which is designed to study the effect of multi-level processes (Hogeweg,

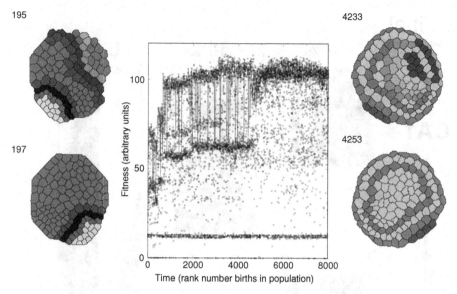

Figure 10.5 Evolutionary fixation of the developmental attractor. The middle panel shows fitness vs. time of the entire quasi-species. The lines connect the individuals which became the shared ancestors of later populations. Up to $t = 4700$ alternative developmental attractors exist and therefore low-fitness individuals may yet become common ancestors. The figures at the sides show examples of alternative attractors of single genotypes. Numbers correspond to rank number as on x axis of central graph. On the left; very early in the simulation, on the right just before the fixation of the high-fitness attractor. Lower figures, low-fitness, upper figures high-fitness morphotype. Note that at all times low-fitness mutants occur. Note also that during fixation of the high-fitness attractor, its fitness temporarily decreases.

2000a, b, 2002). The model consists of (Boolean) gene regulation networks and cells which interact via differential adhesion and local cell signalling, which are defined by the state of the gene network. We evolve gene networks which cause cell differentiation (i.e. unlike the model of Kaneko discussed in above (pp. 179–180), we use an external fitness criterion rather than cell division rate). As a side effect of the cell differentiation intricate morphgenesis may appear.

A phenomenon similar to the 'phenotype-first' effect is observed in this model in the following way:

- Fitness increases in a punctuated manner as is usually the case in systems with non-linear genotype–phenotype mapping (van Nimwegen *et al.*, 1999a). Here, however, a step in maximum fitness may not be accompanied by an increase in average (and median) fitness (see Fig. 10.5).
- In these cases the high-fitness state is just one of the possible outcomes of the developmental process which in the early stages is sensitive to the

exact plane of division. This affects, apart from fitness, gene expression, growth and morphogenesis.

- Eventually evolution stabilises the high-fitness state. This stabilisation increases average/median fitness but not maximum fitness. This is a special case for the evolution towards robustness which is demonstrated in both experiments and in theory (van Nimwegen *et al.*, 1999b) as being a generic property of evolution.

A kind of 'mutational priming' is seen as repeated reinvention of morphotypes during one evolutionary run, or in parallel evolutionary runs:

- Starting with random Boolean networks, the subsequent evolution is extremely sensitive to noise: using a real-time, parallel computer network makes runs entirely non-repeatable, even when we use identical pseudo-random generator seeds, because of time differences.
- After reaching maximum fitness both the 'genotype' (i.e. the fully specified gene regulation network) and the 'transcriptosome' (here defined as the simplified gene regulation network which contains activatable links) continue to change, although the latter, unlike the former, slows down after the plateau is reached.
- The morphology of the ancestor lineage changes only slightly, i.e. the basic cell differentiation pattern remains the same, although sometimes other genes are expressed.
- Most interestingly, mutants which are produced along this 'neutral path' may exhibit strikingly different morphologies from the ancestor lineage. Morphologically similar mutants repeatedly arise at distant evolutionary times.
- Similarly, restarting the evolution process from some intermediate stage also tends to produce such mutants.

We conclude that evolving/evolved gene regulation network incorporates more properties than meet the eye: apart from the phenotype they produce, they organise themselves over evolutionary time so as to contain the potential for well-defined alternatives which become apparent either through mutation, or through regulation.

Discussion and conclusions

The studies reviewed above were all done on different systems, and from a different perspective. As reviewed, they all clearly expound a common result: self-organisation is a powerful mechanism to guide evolutionary dynamics. This has been demonstrated from the viewpoint of population interaction (intraspecific and interspecific) and from the viewpoint of intra-cellular (molecular) dynamics. In both contexts we have seen that oscillatory behaviour paves the way to rich dynamical behaviour which paves the way to evolutionary change Moreover, our results suggest that self-organisation is a necessary prerequisite for the evolution of complex information-processing.

Note that we use a somewhat wider concept of self-organisation than that proposed by Camazine *et al.* (2001) in their volume *Self-Organisation in Biological Systems*, which requires that the self-organisation benefits (i.e. increases the fitness of) the species under consideration. Instead, we require that the self-organisation is essential for 'someone' in the system under consideration. Thus we also exclude patterns that are only observed from the outside, but we do include them as soon as they are 'observed' by (and influence) anyone within the system. One way that observation/influence occurs is through evolution. As our examples have shown, in this way the impact of self-organisation goes well beyond 'mere fitness'. Indeed other factors than fitness determine qualitatively different outcomes of evolutionary processes, as demonstrated.

Our examples considered eco-evolutionary and intracellular cellular dynamics. Examples of behavioural systems in combination with evolution are less well developed as yet. More than a decade ago (Hogeweg, 1988; Hogeweg and Hesper, 1991), when we expounded the TODO principle as a pattern-processing mechanism, and its ability to explain patterns of behaviour that were usually explained by evolutionary optimisation, we speculated that the generated self-organised patterns of behaviour might serve as the pre-pattern on which evolution operates. Our examples indicate that this is indeed to be expected, as we have shown how non-heritable acquired states can guide evolutionary change. Moreover we have shown how versatile, environmentally guided and/or computational sophisticated individual behaviour can evolve. We have only seen the evolution of 'individual-based' diversity in cases where self-organization occurs at other levels of the system as well, i.e. as spatial pattern formation (see also Hogeweg, 1994).

In the introduction we discussed various modes of adaptation and observation of the environment. The discussed model experiments suggest that they are equivalent alternative attractors of evolutionary dynamics.

Acknowledgements

I thank my former students, in particular Maarten Boerlijst, Michiel van Boven, Jan van der Laan, Nick Savill, Ludo Pagie and Stan Marée, for their collaboration. I thank Ben Hesper for his collaboration and long-term support.

References

Ben-Shahar, Y., Robichon, A., Sokolowski, M. B. and Robinson, G. E. (2002). Influence of gene action across different time scales on behavior. *Science* **296**, 741–744.

Beshers, S. N., Huang, Z. Y., Oono, Y. and Robinson, G. E. (2001). Social inhibition and the regulation of temporal polyethism in honey bees. *J. Theoret. Biol.* **213**, 461–479.

Boerlijst, M. A. and Hogeweg, P. (1991a). Spiral wave structure in pre-biotic evolution: hypercycles stable against parasites. *Physica D* **48**, 17–28.

(1991b). Selfstructuring and selection: spiral waves as a substrate for prebiotic evolution. In *Artificial Life II: SFI Studies in the Sciences of Complexity*, vol 10, ed. C. G. Langton. Redwood City, CA: Addison-Wesley, pp. 255–276.

Camazine, S., Deneubourg, J.-L., Franks, N. R. *et al.* (2001). *Self-Organisation in Biological Systems*. Princeton, NJ: Princeton University Press.

Crutchfield, J. P. and Mitchell, M. (1995). The evolution of emergent computation. *Proc. Natl Acad. Sci. USA* **92**, 10742–10746.

Czaran, T. L., Hoekstra, R. F. and Pagie, L. (2002). Chemical warfare between microbes promotes biodiversity. *Proc. Natl Acad. Sci. USA* **99**, 786–790.

Eigen, M. and Schuster, P. (1979). *The Hypercycle: A Principle of Natural Self-organisation*. Berlin: Springer-Verlag.

Ferea, T. L., Botstein, D., Brown, P. O. and Rosenzweig, R. F. (1999). Systematic changes in gene expression patterns following adaptive evolution in yeast. *Proc. Natl Acad. Sci USA* **96**, 9721–9726.

Furusawa, C. and Kaneko, K. (2000). 'Origin of complexity in multicellular organisms. *Phys. Rev. Lett.* **84**, 6130–6133.

(2001). Theory of robustness of irreversible differentiation in a stem cell system: chaos hypothesis. *J. Theoret. Biol.* **209**, 395–416.

Givnish, T. J. and Sytsma, K. J. (1997). *Molecular Evolution and Adaptive Radiation*. Cambridge: Cambridge University Press.

Goldbeter, A. (1996). *Biochemical Oscillations and Cellular Rhythms: The Molecular Basis of Periodic and Chaotic Behaviour*. Cambridge: Cambridge University Press.

Hemelrijk, C. K. (1998). Spatial centrality of dominants without positional preference. In *Artificial Life*, vol. 6, ed. C. Adami, R. K. Belew, H. Kitano and C. E. Taylor. Cambridge, MA: MIT Press, pp. 307–315.

(1999). An individual-oriented model on the emergence of despotic and egalitarian societies. *Proc. Roy. Soc. London B* **266**, 361–369.

(2000a). Towards the integration of social dominance and spatial structure. *Anim. Behav.* **59**, 1035–1048.

(2000b). Self-reinforcing dominance interactions between virtual males and females: hypothesis generation for primate studies. *Adapt. Behav.* **8**, 13–26.

Hogeweg, P. (1988). MIRROR beyond MIRROR, puddles of Life. In *Artificial Life: SFI Studies in the Sciences of Complexity*, ed. C. Langton. Redwood City, CA: Addison-Wesley, pp. 297–315.

(1994). On the potential role of DNA in an RNA world: Pattern generation and information accumulation in replicator systems. *Ber. Bunsengesel Phys. Chem.* **98**, 1135–1139.

(1998). On searching generic properties in non-generic phenomena: an approach to bioinformatic theory formation. In *Artificial Life*, vol. 6, ed. C. Adami, R. K. Belew, H. Kitano and C. E. Taylor. Cambridge, MA: MIT Press, pp. 285–294.

(2000a). Evolving mechanism of morphogenesis: on the interplay between differential adhesion and cell differentiation. *J. Theoret. Biol.* **203**, 317–333.

(2000b). Shapes in the shadow: evolutionary dynamics of morphogenesis. *Artif. Life* **6**, 85–101.

(2002). Computing an organism: on the interface between informatic and dynamic processes. *Biosystems* **64**, 97–109.

Hogeweg, P. and Hesper, B. (1983). The ontogeny of the interaction structure in bumble bee colonies: a MIRROR model. *Behav. Ecol. Sociobiol.* **12**, 271–283.

(1985). Socioinformatic processes: a MIRROR modelling methodology. *J. Theoret. Biol.* **113**, 311–330.

(1991). Evolution as pattern processing: TODO as substrate for evolution. In *From Animals to Animats*, ed. J. A. Meyer and S. W. Wilson. Cambridge, MA: MIT Press, pp. 492–497.

Johnson, C. and Boerlijst, M. C. (2002). Selection at the level of the community: the importance of spatial structure. *Trends Ecol. Evol.* **17**, 83–90.

Johnson, C. and Seinen, I. (2002). Selection for restraint in competetive ability in spatial competing systems. *Proc. Roy. Soc. London B* **269**, 655–663.

Kaneko, K. and Yomo, T. (1997). Isologous diversification: a theory of cell differentiation. *Bull. Math. Biol.* **59**, 139–196.

(2000). Sympatric speciation: compliance with phenotype diversification from a single genotype. *Proc. Roy. Soc. London B* **267**, 2367–2373.

(2002). Genetic diversification through interaction-driven phenotype differentiation. *Evol. Eco. Res.* **4**, 317–350.

Laan, J. D. van der and Hogeweg, P. (1995). Predator–prey coevolution: interactions among different time scales. *Proc. Roy. Soc. London B* **259**, 35–42.

Marée, A. F. M., Panfilov, A. V. and Hogeweg, P. (1999a). Migration and thermotaxis of *Dictyostelium discoideum* slugs, a model study. *J. Theoret. Biol.* **199**, 297–309.

(1999b). Phototaxis during the slug stage of *Dictyostelium discoideum*: a model study. *Proc. Roy. Soc. London B* **266**, 1351–1360.

Maynard Smith, J. and Száthmary, E. (1995). *The Major Transitions in Evolution*. San Francisco, CA: W. H. Freeman.

Nimwegen, E. van, Crutchfield, J. P. and Mitchell, M. (1999a). Statistical dynamics of the Royal Road genetic algorithm. *Theoret. Comput. Sci.* **229**, 41–102.

Nimwegen, E. van, Crutchfield, J. P. and Huynen, M. A. (1999b). Neutral evolution of mutational robustness. *Proc. Natl Acad. Sci. USA* **96**, 9716–9720.

Osborne, K. A., Robichon, A., Burgess, E. *et al.* (1997). Natural behavior polymorphism due to a cGMP-dependent protein kinase of *Drosophila*. *Science* **277**, 834–836.

Pacala, S. W., Gordon, D. M. and Godfray, H. C. J. (1996). Effects of social group size on information transfer and task allocation. *Evol. Ecol.* **10**, 127–165.

Pagie, L. W. P. (1999). Information integration in evolutionary processes. Ph.D. thesis, Utrecht University.

Pagie, L. W. P. and Hogeweg, P. (1999). Colicin diversity: a result of eco-evolutionary dynamics. *J. Theoret. Biol.* **196**, 251–261.

(2000a). Individual- and population-based diversity in restriction-modification systems. *Bull. Math. Biol.* **62**, 759–774.

(2000b). Information integration and red queen dynamics in coevolutionary optimization. In *Proc. 2000 Congr. Evol. Computation*, pp. 797–806.

Pagie, L. W. P. and Mitchell, M. (2002). A comparison of evolutionary and coevolutionary search. *Int. J. Comput. Intell. Applic.* **2**, 53–70.

Post, D. J. van der and Hogeweg, P. (2004). Learning what to eat: studying the interrelationship between learning, grouping and environmental conditions in an artificial world. In *Cellular Automata*, ed. P. M. A. Slott, B. Chopard and A. G. Hoekstra. Berlin: Springer-Verlag, pp. 491–501.

Renger, J. J., Yao, W. D., Sokolowski, M. B. and Wu, C. F. (1999). Neuronal polymorphism among natural alleles of a cGMP-dependent kinase gene, foraging, in *Drosophila. J. Neurosci.* **19**, RC28.

Savill, N. J. and Hogeweg, P. (1997). Evolutionary stagnation due to pattern–pattern interactions in a co-evolutionary predator–prey model. *Artif. Life* **3**, 81–100.

Savill, N. J., Rohani, P. and Hogeweg, P. (1997). Self-reinforcing spatial patterns enslave evolution in a host–parasitoid system. *J. Theoret. Biol.* **188**, 11–20.

Seeley, T. D. (1982). Adaptive significance of the age polyethism schedule in honey bee colonies. *Behav. Ecol. Sociobiol.* **11**, 287–294.

Seeley, T. D. and Kolmes, S. A. (1991). Age polyethism for hive duties in honey bees: illusion or reality. *Ethology* **87**, 284–297.

Sokolowski, M. B., Pereira, H. S. and Hughes, K. (1997). Evolution of foraging behavior in *Drosophila* by density-dependent selection. *Proc. Natl Acad. Sci. USA* **94**, 7373–7377.

VanderMeer, J. (1993). Loose coupling of predator–prey cycles: entrainment, chaos and intermittancy in the classic MacArthur consumer resource equations. *Am. Naturalist* **141**, 687–716.

Index